Primary Child and Adolescent Mental Health

Primary Child and Adolescent Mental Health

A practical guide

VOLUME I

Second Edition

Dr Quentin Spender
Consultant in Child and Adolescent Psychiatry
Wolverhampton City Primary Care Trust
Wolverhampton, UK

Dr Judith Barnsley
Consultant in Child and Adolescent Psychiatry
Dorset Healthcare University NHS Foundation Trust
Poole, UK

Alison Davies
Primary Mental Health Worker
Sussex Partnership NHS Foundation Trust
Chichester, UK

and

Dr Jenny Murphy
Clinical Psychologist
Dorset Healthcare University NHS Foundation Trust
Poole, UK

Radcliffe Publishing
London • New York

Radcliffe Publishing Ltd
33–41 Dallington Street
London
EC1V 0BB
United Kingdom

www.radcliffepublishing.com

Electronic catalogue and worldwide online ordering facility.

First Edition 2001

British Library Cataloguing in Publication Data

A catalogue record for this book is available from the British Library.

ISBN-13: 978 184619 314 9 (box set)
ISBN-13: 978 184619 542 6 (volume I)

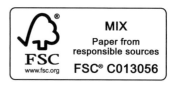

Typeset by KnowledgeWorks Global Ltd, Chennai, India
Printed and bound by TJI Digital, Padstow, Cornwall, UK

Contents

Preface to the second edition

In the decade since the first edition of this book, the way in which mental health services in the United Kingdom are provided to children and adolescents has changed in a number of ways. Although geographical uniformity has proved difficult to achieve, frontline services have been extensively developed to improve the mental health of the under-18 population.

The aim of this book is to give those working at the frontline – the first professionals that a child or parent may meet when asking for help – a practical guide about what to do. The chapters are structured to enable relevant theoretical issues to be summarised simply, followed by detailed suggestions about how to gather relevant information and how to help, leaving referral to specialised services as a last resort.

Our vision is that a whole variety of professionals to whom children or parents may turn for help will have at their fingertips a means of understanding the problems presented, and will be able to offer straightforward ways of helping. Professionals at the frontline need training and advice from more experienced and highly trained colleagues; but we hope this book will also play a role in their professional development and provide an additional source of support, either as a component of learning or as a resource for teaching.

It would be foolhardy not to acknowledge some of the difficulties inherent in providing a universal Child and Adolescent Mental Health Service (CAMHS) that can meet everyone's needs. These barriers include the following.

➤ *Agency cooperation* – Using the broadest definition of CAMHS, services are provided and professionals employed by not only the National Health Service but also by Educational and Social Care organisations; others play a role, such as the youth criminal justice system, substance misuse services and counselling charities. A single child may have contact with a bewildering array of different organisations and individuals, making effective cooperation between them a significant challenge.

➤ *Management issues* – The joint management of Education and Social Care, and the appointment of jointly funded Commissioners, has been introduced to help coordinate the main involved agencies. There remains tremendous variation in management structures. Considering now the narrow definition of CAMHS, specialised services may be part of Mental Health Trusts, Primary Care Trusts or Trusts providing hospital paediatric care. Within these Trusts, specialised CAMHS may be in a directorate with a variety of bedfellows, for instance: adult mental health; adult learning difficulty; community paediatrics; hospital paediatrics; health visiting; school nursing; and many others. Some Trusts favour medics in managerial roles such as that of CAMHS Clinical Director; some Trusts prefer non-clinicians for service management roles; others prefer clinicians such as nurses, psychologists or social workers for both clinical and service management roles.

➤ This variation in management structures is part of the *'postcode lottery'*, meaning that services may be available in one area but not another, and that *where* the child and family live may be as much a factor in determining what help is available as the skill-mix of professionals. Another component of this is that areas of deprivation have higher per capita funding, but in relatively affluent areas, a higher proportion of the population in need may present for help, with the result that services may paradoxically be more stretched in more affluent areas. This can be exacerbated by the cost of housing contributing to difficulties in recruiting staff. The independent sector is just as patchy in its provision (perhaps more). Added to all this is the variation in the four countries of the UK: England, Scotland, Wales and Northern Ireland. We have not attempted in this book to do justice to this, but have stuck to what we know, which is our own practice within three different regions of England: we cannot claim with our limited joint experience to understand the range of service provision within even *one* country.

➤ *Service lacunae* (gaps in what is provided) have persisted, despite a variety of attempts to make services more uniform, such as the National Service Framework[1] and the establishment of a peer-reviewing system.[2] An example is the service received by children with learning difficulties and their families, which is still extremely patchy and highly variable.

➤ *Funding issues* – It is beyond the scope of this book to present the arguments about the inequitable share of the funding cake allocated to under-18s compared to other age groups, or mental health problems compared to other categories of ill health. Killers such as cancer, heart disease or premature birth are more likely to get the sort of publicity that mobilises political will. Some have described CAMHS as the 'Cinderella of Cinderellas'. Periods of investment tend to be followed by periods of renewed financial stringency. Joint commissioning arrangements may not be able to prevent huge sums being spent on highly specialised provision for a small number of individuals, thus stifling investment in small-scale outpatient teams: a larger scale preventative approach may be necessary for this.

➤ *Customer confusion* – All of this variation may leave parents very confused about how best to access help for their child. Professionals may also be confused about who is best placed to deliver the best help at the best time: the professional who first sees the child may be chosen more by accident than by any logical process. Some acronyms (abbreviations) may add to the overall confusion. We give here a selection:

— ABE   Achieving Best Evidence
— ASBO   Antisocial Behaviour Order
— ASSIST   Asylum Seeker Support Initiative Short Term
— BESD   Behavioural, Educational and Social Difficulties
— BEST   Behavioural and Educational Support Team
— BOSS   Business Opportunity Sourcing Service
— BPD   Borderline Personality Disorder
— BPD   Bipolar Disorder
— BPD   Broncho-Pulmonary Dysplasia
— BPS   British Psychological Society
— CAF   Common Assessment Framework
— CAFE   Child and Adolescent Faculty Executive
— CAP   Child and Adolescent Psychiatry
— CORC   CAMHS Outcome Research Consortium
— CPD   Continuing Professional Development
— CPD   Continuous Peritoneal Dialysis
— CPS   Crown Prosecution Service
— CRB   Criminal Records Bureau
— DAT   Drug and Alcohol Team
— DAT   Drug Action Team
— DCSF   Department for Children, Schools and Families
— DNA   Did Not Arrive
— DNA   Deoxyribonucleic acid
— DoH   Department of Health
— DTO   Detention and Training Order
— EBD   Educational and Behavioural Difficulties
— EBPD   Emerging Borderline Personality Disorder
— E2E   Entry to Employment
— FAST   Family Advice and Support Team
— FIP   Family Intervention Project
— FRT   Family Resource Team
— GAP   Guideline Appraisal Panel
— HAVOC   Having an Alternative View of Crime
— HMYOI   Her Majesty's Young Offender Institution
— IRS worker   Integrated Resettlement Support worker
— ISP   Initial Supervision Plan
— ISSP   Intensive Supervision and Surveillance Programme
— JAR   Joint Area Review
— KYPE   Keeping Young People Engaged
— LAC   Looked-After Children
— LD   Learning Difficulty
— MAPPA   Multi-Agency Public Protection Arrangements
— MAST   Multi-Agency Support Team
— MHPW   Mental Health and Psychological Wellbeing
— MLD   Moderate Learning Difficulty

— NEET   Not in Education, Employment or Training
— NHS   National Health Service
— NICE   National Institute for Health and Clinical
                Excellence
— OFSTED   Office for Standards in Education
— OoH   Out of Hours
— PAYP   Positive Activities for Young People
— PCAMHW   Primary Child and Adolescent Mental Health Worker
— PCSO   Police Community Service Officer
— PCT   Primary Care Trust
— PDP   Personal Development Plan
— PHEW   Psychological Health and Emotional Wellbeing
— PMHW   Primary Mental Health Worker
— PREMs   Patient-Reported Experience Measures
— PROMs   Patient-Reported Outcome Measures
— PRU   Pupil Referral Unit
— PTSD   Post Traumatic Stress Disorder
— PSA   Parenting Support Adviser
— PSR   Pre-Sentence Report
— RAP   Recurrent Abdominal Pain
— RAP   Resource Allocation Panel
— RAP   Resettlement and Aftercare Provision
— RoH   Risk of Harm
— SENCo   Special Educational Needs Coordinator
— SIG   Special Interest Group
— SIPS   Social Inclusion and Pupil Support
— SLA   Service Level Agreement
— SLD   Severe Learning Difficulty
— SMART   Specific, Measurable, Achievable, Realistic and
                Time-bounded
— SPP   Senior Parenting Practitioner
— SSIW   Social Services Inspectorate for Wales
— TAC   Team Around the Child
— TaMHS   Targeted Mental Health in Schools
— TPU   Teenage Pregnancy Unit
— VLO   Victim Liaison Officer
— WPI   Wales Programme for Improvement
— YADAS   Young Adults' Drug and Alcohol Service
— YIP   Youth Inclusion Programme
— YISP   Youth Inclusion Support Panel
— YJB   Youth Justice Board
— YOI   Young Offender's Institution
— YOIS   Youth Offending Information System
— YOT   Youth Offending Team
— … and many others.

Another change since the first edition of this book is the increasing availability of protocols and guidelines developed to reduce the risks inherent in any dabbling with other people's mental health – and the variability of clinical approach inevitable in a multidisciplinary field. Some are local, others are national, in particular the Scottish Intercollegiate Guideline Network (SIGN)[3] guidelines in Scotland and the National Institute for Health and Clinical Excellence (NICE)[4] guidelines for the whole UK. These aim to make clinical practice more evidence-based and uniform, and should in theory reduce the postcode lottery.

Other developments such as leaflets,[5] information sheets,[6] websites[7] and charities[8] have aimed at reducing the confusion for families of knowing which profession they should go to when, and the confusion for professionals about whether they are duplicating others' work, or alternatively allowing families to fall into the gaps between services. Various ways of combining professionals from different disciplines into teams who are more coordinated, or more convenient for families, or more convenient for agencies, have been devised (see some of the acronyms above), but there seems to be a remarkable lack of uniformity. The Common Assessment Framework[9] is an attempt to save professionals in different agencies from carrying out repeated initial assessments that ask all the same questions: once done by one agency, it should be shared electronically with others who need to be involved. The use of Electronic Health Records is already common in Health Centres, and is due to spread to specialist CAMHS as we write this edition. We anticipate some difficulties including all the information gathered by specialist CAMHS in electronic form – not least because of concerns about who will access the information.

Just as the expectations placed on professionals working in all levels of CAMHS have changed in a decade, so have the lives of young people been transformed by readily available internet access. Social contact can now take place without anyone leaving their rooms. Cyber-bullying and internet grooming (leading to sexual abuse) have added new dimensions to the hazards of adolescent relationships. Whereas previously we might have worried whether we should allow a parent to show us her daughter's diary without permission, we may now be worried about whether to look at a personal blog, and how we should respond to what we may find there. Similarly, whilst there is much helpful information on the Internet, young people can also access unhelpful sites such as pro-anorexia and pro-suicide websites that compound their despair and undermine the help they may be offered or at least need.

One change that has particularly affected the target audience for this book is the advent, at least in some areas, of the Primary Child and Adolescent Mental Health Worker, variously abbreviated as PCAMHW or PMHW. This specialism was just being developed as the first edition was being published. The initial idea for the book (which we must credit to Professor Peter Hill) was as a source of practical information for those working in primary care – the case examples were written with General Practitioners in mind – but GPs may have been only a small proportion of the book's readership. Professor Hill was also part of the group that developed[10] the idea of the Four Tier system and the Primary Child and Adolescent Mental Health Worker (for further details *see* Chapter 1: Context).

The first edition seems to have been devoured by a variety of professionals doing Tier 1 and Tier 2 work, and we hope this edition will cater more overtly for these groups. We have shifted the emphasis to make the book suitable for any profession to whom the Primary Child and Adolescent Mental Health Worker consults. We hope the book will enable frontline practitioners (Tier 1 or universal services) to catch child mental health conditions at an early stage so that interventions can be provided without having to wait for specialised services (Tier 3 or targeted services) to become involved. The authorship, instead of being a mixture of Child and Adolescent Psychiatrists and GPs, is now a mixture of Child and Adolescent Psychiatrists and Primary Child and Adolescent Mental Health Workers.

Rather than tinker with the first edition, we have rewritten the whole book, reorganising some of the chapter structure, but keeping the more successful chapters while updating them. We have persisted in our strategy of breaking-up the text by liberal use of bullet points, tables, case examples, summary boxes (including 'Practice Points' and 'Alarm Bells') and figures. The most striking change is perhaps the first main section of the book (Chapters 2 to 4), which emphasises our developmental approach by describing the differences between three important development stages: pre-school, middle childhood and adolescence. In particular, the chapter on middle childhood contains much of the content of the first chapter in the first edition, which was entitled 'Assessment'. We have also changed the title, to reflect the change in emphasis.

A note on terminology: We have alternated the female and male pronoun when talking about an unspecified child (or parent). We are aware there are various definitions of 'children' (for instance: under-13, Gillick incompetent, under-16 or under-18); 'adolescents' (12–25 being perhaps the most inclusive); and 'young people' (for instance, 16- and 17-year-olds, 11–19 or seven to 25). But we have used these terms colloquially, without attempting to stick to one definition. We have also used the terms 'parent' and 'carer' interchangeably (so as to avoid the cumbersome phrase 'parent or carer'). We have tried to keep abbreviations to a minimum, but have allowed ourselves to use a few, such as: 'CAMHS' for Child and Adolescent Mental Health Services; 'ADHD' for Attention-Deficit/Hyperactivity Disorder; GCSEs for General Certificate of Secondary Education exams; and 'DVDs' for Digital Versatile Discs.

A note on case examples: We have pursued a policy of peppering the text liberally with these, in order to break up the text, maintain clinical relevance and keep things interesting. The case examples vary in their origins: some are based on a single case, with enough details altered to make the identity unrecognisable to anyone but the child and family; some incorporate details of more than one case; and some are fictionalised on the basis of our clinical experience (so effectively incorporating the details of many cases).

We hope that our labours will enable our readers to improve the mental health and emotional well-being of children throughout the United Kingdom, and possibly elsewhere.

Quentin Spender
Judith Barnsley
Alison Davies
Jenny Murphy
April 2011

REFERENCES

1 www.dh.gov.uk/en/Publicationsandstatistics/Publications/PublicationsPolicyAnd Guidance/DH_4089114
2 www.rcpsych.ac.uk/crtu/centreforqualityimprovement/qinmaccamhs.aspx
3 www.sign.ac.uk
4 www.nice.org.uk
5 www.rcpsych.ac.uk
6 CAMHS Evidence Based Practice Unit. *Choosing What's Best For You: what scientists have found helps children and young people who are sad, worried or troubled.* London: CAMHS publications; July 2007. Available at: www.annafreud.org/ebpu (accessed 20 March 2011).
7 www.mentalhealth.org.uk
8 www.youngminds.org.uk
9 www.education.gov.uk/childrenandyoungpeople/strategy/integratedworking/caf/a0068957/the-caf-process
10 Health Advisory Service. *Together We Stand: the commissioning, role and management of child and adolescent mental health services.* London: HMSO; 1995.

About the authors

Dr Quentin Spender, Consultant in Child and Adolescent Psychiatry, Wolverhampton City Primary Care Trust, Wolverhampton, UK

Dr Judith Barnsley, Consultant in Child and Adolescent Psychiatry, Dorset Healthcare University NHS Foundation Trust, Poole, UK

Alison Davies, Primary Mental Health Worker, Sussex Partnership NHS Foundation Trust, Chichester, UK

Dr Jenny Murphy, Clinical Psychologist, Dorset Healthcare University NHS Foundation Trust, Poole, UK

Acknowledgements

This book germinated from an idea that we must credit to Professor Emeritus Peter Hill, who wanted to fashion a companion volume to the same publisher's *The Child Surveillance Handbook*,[1] of which he was an initial co-author. Along with our own changing co-authorship, we have benefited from the direct or indirect input of the following: Rosemarie Berry, Chrissy Boardman, Teri Boutwood, Nina Bunce, Anna Calver, Esther Crawley, David Candy, Steve Clarke, David Rex, Moira Doolan, Danya Glaser, Gill Goodwillie, Sue Horobin, Amelia Kerswell, Karen King, Sebastian Kraemer, Karen Majors, Rebecca Park, Joanna Pearse, Nigel Speight, Anne Stewart and Wendy Woodhouse. We would also like to thank the children and families whom we have all seen in our clinical work: they have taught us so much, and many of them have provided us with the stories for our case examples.

Note

1 First edition published in 1990, second edition published in 1994 and third edition published in 2009. Hall D, Williams J, Elliman D. *The Child Surveillance Handbook*. 3rd ed. London and New York: Radcliffe Publishing; 2009.

PART 1

Overview

CHAPTER 1

The context for provision of Child and Adolescent Mental Health Services

A DEFINITION OF CHILD MENTAL HEALTH

Mental health in children and young people has been defined as having the following components:[1]

➤ a capacity to enter into and sustain mutually satisfying personal relationships
➤ a continuing progression of psychological development
➤ an ability to play and to learn so that attainments are appropriate for age and intellectual level
➤ a developing moral sense of right and wrong
➤ the degree of psychological distress and maladaptive behaviour is within normal limits for the child's age and context.

Additional aspects of emotional well-being include the following:

➤ a capacity to use and enjoy solitude
➤ empathy and awareness of others' feelings
➤ continuing emotional, intellectual and spiritual development
➤ becoming able to learn and benefit from setbacks or problems.

In the words of one young person reporting to the 2008 UK Child and Adolescent Mental Health Services (CAMHS) review panel, which will be quoted extensively in this chapter: 'It doesn't mean being happy all the time but it does mean being able to cope with things.'[2]

Child mental health problems are therefore difficulties or disabilities in these areas that may arise from any number of congenital, constitutional, environmental, family or illness factors. Such problems have two components: *firstly*, the presenting features are outside the normal range for the child's developmental age, intellectual level and culture ('deviance' – with a statistical more than a sociological meaning); and *secondly*, the child or others are suffering from the dysfunction ('impairment'). Or to put it in a nutshell:

Disorder = deviance plus impairment.

There is no mental health disorder unless both aspects are present.

THE ORGANISATION OF SERVICES

Children's mental health needs, in the broadest sense, are met by a multitude of people: firstly, and most obviously, by their parents (or carers), other relatives and friends; but also by a variety of professionals, from those who look after the baby in hospital, the toddler in nursery, the child in school and the adolescent in youth clubs to the various professionals working in multidisciplinary teams that we will call 'specialist CAMHS'.

The Four-Tier model

This broad approach to service delivery was the basis for the Health Advisory Service Report 'Together We Stand',[3] which provided a new way of thinking about how CAMHS can be organised. The authors of the report[4] proposed two new concepts: the *Four-Tier* system and the ***primary mental health worker*** (PMHW or PCAMHW). These concepts can still give rise to endless confusion and debate, although their description in the original document is fairly clear. Part of the reason for the confusion is that services have developed in very different ways in different parts of the United Kingdom, so that people whose job titles are the same may do very different things, and the same service may be provided in different areas by people with different training or job titles. Teams of people working together to help children, young people and their families may have a variety of different names. Examples include:
➤ 'Team Around the Child'
➤ 'Behavioural and Educational Support Team'
➤ 'Multi-Agency Support Team'
➤ 'Social Inclusion Team'
➤ 'Integrated Service Delivery Areas'
➤ 'Primary Care Behaviour Service'
➤ 'Children's Emotional Health and Wellbeing Service'
➤ 'Targeted Mental Health in Schools' team
➤ and many others.

Our attempts in this book to explain these concepts will inevitably fall foul of such geographical variability in the way that services and teams are named – as well as the frequent major changes that are made to the ways in which services are delivered, particularly with each new government.

Figure 1.1 attempts to clarify the Four-Tier model, but with the strong caveat that the exact placement within the diagram of each profession may seem appropriate only in some areas.

The traditional threefold division of services was into *primary* care (who refer onto) *secondary* or specialist care (who refer onto) *tertiary* care – even more specialist care – traditionally in the local teaching hospital.

In the fourfold model, Tier 1 practitioners are those working in universal services, such as primary care, schools or youth clubs. These professionals are not primarily trained as mental health specialists – but mental health and emotional

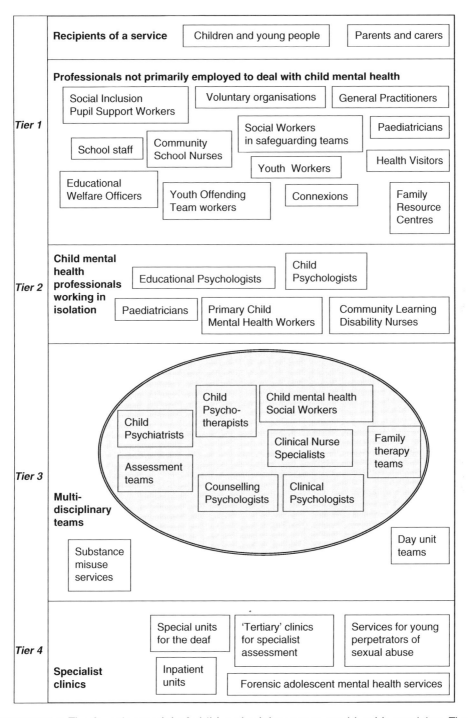

FIGURE 1.1 The four tier model of child and adolescent mental health provision. The oval represents specialist CAMHS

well-being is increasingly seen as everyone's business. Their role includes: promoting mental health; providing general advice, support and treatment for less severe problems; helping to identify problems early; and referring on to more specialised services.[5] An example of this sort of work is given in Box 1.1.

BOX 1.1 Case Example

Sandra, aged four years, is referred to her health visitor by her nursery school because she is having episodes of rage during which she goes blue and appears to stop breathing. The health visitor checks that Sandra's mother, Janet, has given consent to the referral and then visits her at home, while Sandra is there, to discuss the concerns. She then visits the nursery school to talk to the staff and following this she reviews the situation with a local primary mental health worker.

The health visitor and primary mental health worker have little difficulty establishing that these episodes, which happen at home as well as at the nursery school, are blue breath-holding attacks. Although there are no concerning features in the history, Janet remains anxious about the breath-holding attacks and so the health visitor arranges for a general practitioner's appointment, where a thorough history, examination and explanation provides Janet with some reassurance.

The health visitor then gives Janet the behavioural management advice contained in Chapter 18 of this book on Breath-holding. She reinforces this advice with further telephone support and a home visit six weeks later.

At this follow-up, the attacks have substantially reduced and Janet is much more confident about managing the behaviour.

Tiers 2 and 3 include the traditional narrowly defined 'specialist CAMHS' service in the oval, which is part of secondary care. A referral from Tier 1 is usually necessary to allow a child or family to have access to it. Tier 2 is uni-disciplinary and Tier 3 multi-disciplinary. Tier 2 professionals have specific mental health training. They may support service delivery at Tier 1 by carrying out assessment, treatment, consultation or training. Tier 3 teams usually offer a specialised service to those with more severe, complex and persistent disorders. Confusion sometimes arises with this model because the same professional may work in Tier 2 and Tier 3 in the same day: she may be working in isolation in the morning, but in collaboration with others in the afternoon. The nature of multidisciplinary working is also a little ambiguous: does it require the young person or family to be seen by more than one professional, or is it sufficient for the case referred to be discussed by several professionals for the approach to be considered multidisciplinary?

Tier 4 services are more highly specialised, are roughly equivalent to tertiary care, and usually require a referral from Tiers 2 or 3. Most serve a larger area than the referring Tier 2/3 services.

It is debatable whether there are any other professionals in Tiers 2 or 3 who work outside the oval: educational psychologists used to work regularly in specialist CAMHS teams, but now seldom do; however, many are now part of separate multidisciplinary teams centred around a school or group of schools. Day units may be staffed by the same professionals who work for part of their week in specialist CAMHS teams. Individuals within the oval may work partly in conjunction with other team members (Tier 3) and partly on their own (Tier 2), so may effectively be part of both tiers. Some Tier 4 teams may work in relative isolation, so seem more like services at Tier 2 or Tier 3 level: for instance, substance misuse teams.

A development of this Four-Tier model has been an extra tier (not included on our diagram) between specialist outpatient (Tier 3) and inpatient (Tier 4) services, often referred to as Tier 3+ or Tier 3½. These sub-teams may take various forms, including crisis intervention teams managed by a Tier 3 service or outreach teams managed by a Tier 4 service. They are thought to lessen the number and duration of costly inpatient admissions, and therefore more than save what they cost.

One of the underlying principles of this model is that children's mental health needs should be met at the lowest tier possible. This book can be seen as part of this general trend to empower a wider range of professionals in fulfilling the maxim that child mental health and emotional well-being is everybody's business.[6]

Uni-disciplinary versus multidisciplinary working

There is no research evidence we are aware of to prove that multidisciplinary working has a better (or worse) outcome than uni-disciplinary working, but clinical experience suggests that straightforward cases can be helped effectively by a skilled worker from almost any relevant background, whereas more complex cases require the input of more than one discipline. To insist that all cases referred for help should have multidisciplinary input, or worse still multi-agency input, is unnecessarily expensive. A more flexible approach that is needs-led by the individual child or family may be more cost-effective.[7] Some would go further and point out a potential risk that the more professionals involved with a child, the less effective they are all likely to be in helping the child and family: but it may be simply that the child has complex needs of a sort that are not easy to remedy by one professional, but which draw in a large number of different professionals. In this case, cooperation is essential, as opposed to duplication or working in contrary directions, and may require the agreed appointment of a lead professional, a key worker or a care-coordinator, as well as regular (and very costly) multi-professional meetings (called in some places the Team Around the Child). A Common Assessment Framework meeting may kick-start this process.[8]

Paediatric mental health

The provision of mental health services is not confined to mental health practitioners: paediatricians, both in hospital and even more so in the community, manage a great many mental health problems, often without much support from overstretched specialist CAMHS services (Tier 2/3). These may include mental health problems experienced by:

➤ children with disability, particularly neurological disability or sensory impairment
➤ children who have been abused
➤ looked-after children
➤ children who present primarily with physical symptoms that are subsequently found to be indicators of an underlying mental health problem
➤ autistic spectrum disorders
➤ ADHD.

Some families may prefer to see a paediatrician for such problems, as they perceive this as less stigmatising than attending a mental health service. In Figure 1.1, we have placed paediatricians in both Tier 1 and Tier 2, but some may soon be within Tier 3, due to a training programme in paediatric mental health that has been developed while we wrote this edition; and some paediatric neurologists may be involved in Tier 4 neuro-psychiatric assessment teams. This illustrates that arguments about which tier a particular person is working at are likely to be unhelpful. Another pitfall of the Four-Tier model is the professional snobbery that sometimes develops between the tiers, on the assumption that the higher a tier in which a professional works, the more skilled she must be. So staff in inpatient units may look down on outpatient teams, whose members may in turn look down upon uni-disciplinary working – which may in fact be the most challenging of all and require the most skill – not least because a sole professional is doing it.

The Four-Tier model is simply one way of understanding how services are organised; an alternative model, which some may see as more user-friendly, is described below.

The concept of the primary mental health worker

To reinforce the development of child mental health provision in Tier 1 settings and link this to existing Tier 2 and 3 provisions, the Health Advisory Service proposed the new job title of 'primary mental health worker', who works in Tier 2. This would not be a new discipline, but merely a new role. Professionals filling this role could include clinical nurse specialists, social workers, child psychologists or any other child mental health professional with sufficient training to work as a generalist in a variety of settings. It was assumed their role would include:

➤ direct assessment and treatment for mild to moderate difficulties
➤ consultation and advice to members of Tier 1 services
➤ referral when necessary to the local specialist CAMHS (Tier 2/3 service)
➤ providing child mental health training to Tier 1 service providers.

And so it has turned out (roughly), with the inevitable large geographical variation in management structures and job descriptions.

An alternative model

The Four-Tier model is merely a way of looking at existing services and helping to organise them, so it is not susceptible to randomised controlled trials, as some

TABLE 1.1 Universal, targeted and specialist services

Universal services	Work with all children and young people. They promote and support mental health and psychological well-being through the environment they create and the relationships they have with children and young people. They include early years providers and settings such as childminders and nurseries, schools, colleges, youth services and primary healthcare services such as GPs, midwives and health visitors.
Targeted services	Are engaged to work with children and young people who have specific needs – for example, learning difficulties or disabilities, school attendance problems, family difficulties, physical illness or behaviour difficulties. Within this group of services we also include CAMHS delivered to targeted groups of children, such as those in care.
Specialist services	Work with children and young people with complex, severe and/ or persistent needs, reflecting the needs rather than necessarily the 'specialist' skills required to meet those needs. This includes CAMHS at Tiers 3 and 4 of the conceptual framework (though there is overlap here as some Tier 3 services could also be included in the 'targeted' category). It also includes services across education, social care and youth offending that work with children and young people with the highest levels of need – for example, in pupil referral units (PRUs), special schools, children's homes, intensive foster care and other residential or secure settings.

have suggested. While very helpful in guiding thinking about the development of CAMHS in the broadest sense, it has led to frequent misunderstandings and unproductive debates about who fits into what tier at which time of day.

A more recent model is shown in Table 1.1.[9] This divides services into universal, targeted and specialist, thereby in some ways reverting to the old primary/secondary/tertiary model, but extending it well beyond health. It overcomes some of the definitional conflicts inherent in the Four-Tier model. It remains to be seen whether this model will increase clarity and reduce confusion (as intended) – or will in time become susceptible to the same drift in meaning and inter-professional rivalry that has sabotaged the clarity of the Four-Tier model. One potential confusion is that so-called 'specialist' services are not necessarily the most specialised in terms of professional training but *are* specialised in terms of the multiple needs of the children they select to treat. It might make more sense to call them 'multi-needs services' or 'multi-professional services'.

What children, young people and families want

'What children, young people and their families and carers want is often quite simple. They told us they want consistent relationships with people who can help and to be treated with dignity and respect.'[10] This is expanded in Table 1.2:[11]

TABLE 1.2 How to make services more effective: themes defined by children and carers

Awareness	There should be more awareness in children's centres, schools, colleges and primary care health centres about: • mental health • how to promote it • how to deal sensitively with issues that arise.
Trust	There should be opportunities to build a trusting relationship with a known member of staff in schools, so that problems can be shared and discussed.
	There should be regular contact with the same staff in targeted and specialist services.
	There should be clarity over confidentiality arrangements.
Accessibility	Services should be in convenient places.
	Information and advice should be available in a range of relevant formats and media.
	There should be a single point of entry to specialist mental health services.
	Services should be age-appropriate.
Communication	Whichever service you are dealing with, it is important to feel listened to and given individual attention.
	The language used by staff should be straightforward, with no technical jargon.
Involvement	You should be valued for the insight and experience you bring.
	There should be opportunities to discuss what services and interventions are available.
Support when it's needed	Services should be available when the need first arises, not just when things reach crisis point.
	Services should stay in touch after support or treatment has finished and follow up any problems.
Holistic approach	Services should think about you as an individual – for example, providing help with practical issues and addressing your physical health as well as your mental health

It's not all up to health

The old threefold model of primary, secondary and tertiary care assumed that everything is provided by health, which may still be the case in the specialities of surgery, but is no longer the case for children's mental health. Youth offending teams, for instance, may include only one health employee (or in some cases none); while specialist teams for assessing and treating young perpetrators of sexual abuse may be financed and staffed by a charity such as the National Society for the Prevention of Cruelty to Children. Youth workers can provide valuable input for young people who may not feel comfortable with the nature of other helping services.

Connexions was set up as an extension of the Careers Advisory Service, but its expanded remit can include sorting out many mental health issues, especially for young people with learning difficulties, or those who, for other reasons, do not fit into readily available educational or employment opportunities. There are many other examples of organisations that contribute to children's emotional health and well-being: steps have been taken to ensure that all have a 'common core' of training.[12] In particular, education and social care contribute a large component of overall mental health provision.

Education

In schools, support for individual children is invaluable, either in the form of someone a child can talk to if she needs, or special needs help. Group or class-room initiatives are also important, either as part of lessons in personal, social and health education, or preferably as part of a whole school prioritisation of pastoral care. Teaching staff and learning support assistants within the school may be supported by local partnership teams centred on a cluster of schools. These teams may have a variety of names (*see* the bullet-point list on page 4). They can include a variety of professionals: educational psychologists; specialist advisory teachers; social workers; school nurses; mental health workers with links to Tier 3 CAMHS; educational welfare officers; social inclusion workers; and representatives from youth services, children's centres, the police or voluntary organisations. These may form a 'virtual team', with members who are based in different teams on different sites, or a real team, with co-located offices. Coordination of input from different agencies may be a challenge, and may require different sorts of solutions in different localities. Special schools may need more specialist input. Meeting the mental health needs of 14–19 year olds may result in particular difficulties for sixth-form colleges and Connexions, not least because of the variable age cut-offs of different agencies.

BOX 1.2 Case Example

> Robert, aged 14 years, is having difficulty managing in school due to his behaviour. He has been to his local specialist CAMHS service for assessment of possible ADHD, but has refused a trial of medication, and says he does not want to return for any more appointments.
>
> His father left home when he was three years old after a period of domestic violence. His mother has two younger children by a different father, who has also left the family home. She had a difficult relationship with her own mother, but Robert has always got on well with his maternal grandfather and one of his maternal uncles.
>
> At school, he gets into frequent fights and is often sent out of the classroom for being disruptive. He responds well to small-group or individual tuition in the Learning Support Unit (Special Needs Department), but is getting low grades for most subjects, especially those involving literacy skills. He is however good at physical education and craft, design and technology. He has recently been given three short-term

exclusions, for a combination of fighting with other pupils and swearing at teachers. His mother is concerned that most of Robert's friends seem to be involved in minor criminal activities and possibly drug use (which Robert denies).

The special needs coordinator is concerned that Robert will be permanently excluded, so, with his mother's permission, seeks advice from the primary mental health worker. Together, they agree that the special needs coordinator will approach her local partnership team for further advice and in particular the social inclusion worker. The social inclusion worker meets with Robert and his mother: he tries to focus on Robert's strengths rather than his problems. He gets Robert onto a local activity scheme, which involves Robert in after-school and Saturday morning activities, including a martial arts class, skateboarding, a drama group and a guitar workshop. Robert makes a good relationship with a particular youth worker, who manages to encourage Robert to establish a more pro-social group of friends, so that he keeps out of trouble with the police. The special needs coordinator enrols Robert at the beginning of Year 10 into college courses, each for one day per week, in motor mechanics and carpentry, both of which he enjoys. He is allowed to reduce the number of GCSEs he is enrolled for.

Over the next two years, Robert narrowly manages to avoid permanent school exclusion, although he still has difficulties managing classroom situations with particular teachers, and has to spend about half of his remaining three days in school in the Learning Support Unit. He gets a D grade in Maths GCSE, and with support from his Connexions worker, continues at college on a carpentry course while taking his English GCSE re-sit. He has some difficulty getting an apprenticeship, but eventually finds one with a relative. Although he still clashes with his mother about his late bedtimes and untidy room, she is pleased about the friends he has made.

Higher levels of organisation

The work of different agencies needs coordination. In England, this can be provided locally by children's trusts or strategic partnerships, but there seems to be ample scope for confusion about which of many intermediate management structures is responsible for what, perhaps partly because there are two government ministries mainly responsible (the Department of Health and the Department for Education – previously the Department of Children, Schools and Families). Variations in commissioning arrangements and funding streams, both geographically and in time cycles, can make it difficult at times to implement the hard-won agreements made at strategic planning meetings. More effective coordination at a national level may be provided by the National Advisory Council, which aims to hold government, children's trusts and commissioners to account in implementing the conclusions of the National CAMHS review.

Wales, Scotland and Northern Ireland have different structures for coordinating provision.

THE BROADER CONTEXT: INEQUALITY

Any textbook such as this is in danger of giving the impression that children's mental health is remediable only by the measures described herein. It is therefore worth emphasising, as others have done,[13] that measures of a different nature may be equally – or perhaps more – important. These are concerned with remedying the social and economic context in which mental health issues arise. Indeed, some argue[14] that these are the main determinants of international differences in mental health, such as those highlighted in a 2007 UNICEF report.[15] A recent British report was commissioned to review the evidence and make recommendations.[16] A selection of issues raised may serve to illustrate how much more is relevant to children's mental health and well-being than we could hope to cover in this book.

➤ Children from disadvantaged backgrounds are more likely to begin primary school with lower personal, social and emotional development and communication, language and literacy skills than their peers.[17] These children are also at significantly increased risk of developing conduct disorders that could lead to difficulties in all areas of their lives, including educational attainment, relationships and longer-term mental health. There are clear *socioeconomic gradients* in all these factors.

➤ Even the best primary schools struggle with an intake of children who lack '*school readiness*', that is, those whose behaviour stops them from learning or who lack the necessary communication and social interaction skills. Cost-effectiveness analysis of early literacy interventions shows a significant return on investment: for instance, the 'Every Child a Reader' programme could offer a return of more than £17 in the next 31 years for every £1 spent now, based on the estimated costs of problems associated with continuing poor literacy such as truancy and poor employment prospects.

➤ *Early intervention* through intensive home visiting programmes during and after pregnancy can be effective in improving the health, well-being and self-sufficiency of low-income, young first-time parents and their children. An example of this being successfully applied in the UK is the Family Nurse Partnership programme[18] in Tower Hamlets, East London.[19] Proven benefits from home visiting, to both mother and child, include:
   — improvements in the mother's prenatal health
   — improved parenting skills
   — greater involvement of fathers
   — improved child development
   — reduced behavioural problems
   — fewer injuries to children
   — a reduction in child maltreatment[20]
   — improvements in school readiness
   — fewer arrests of children when they reach adolescence
   — fewer subsequent pregnancies (in the mother)
   — increased maternal employment
   — improved maternal mental health and social functioning.

➤ High-quality *preschool programmes* (nursery schooling) can improve children's self-esteem and behaviour. Better outcomes include:
  — a higher rate of subsequent adult employment
  — fewer crimes committed
  — being more likely to complete school
  — having higher earnings.
➤ *Bad housing conditions*: including homelessness, temporary accommodation, overcrowding, insecurity, and housing in poor physical condition – constitute a risk to health, including mental health: children in bad housing conditions are more likely to have mental health problems such as anxiety and depression, experience long-term disability and have delayed cognitive development. These adverse outcomes reflect both the direct impact of the housing and the associated material deprivation.
➤ Living close to areas of *green space* – parks, woodland and other open spaces – can improve health, regardless of social class.
  — Green spaces have been associated with improved mental health and reduced stress levels, plus an increased ability to face problems.
  — The presence of green space near the home encourages social contact and integration.
  — Exercising outside can have more positive mental health benefits than exercise of other kinds.
  — Marking school playgrounds with designs that stimulate active games is associated with a 20% long-term improvement in physical activity.
  — A natural play environment at school also helps to reduce bullying, increase creative play, improve concentration and increase self-esteem.
➤ Availability of *healthy food*, and in particular fresh produce, is often worse in deprived areas due to the mix of shops that tend to locate in these neighbourhoods. For instance, McDonald's outlets in England and Scotland are four times more concentrated in the most deprived areas than in the least deprived areas. Low-income groups are more likely to consume fat spreads, non-diet soft drinks, meat dishes, pizzas, processed meats, whole milk and table sugar than the better-off.

We have included a chapter on diet and exercise, but have not included chapters on how to help children who start school with socio-economic disadvantage to catch up; town planning; or how to lobby politicians.

Young people who are disengaged[21]

A proportion of secondary school pupils may not find what is taught in the classroom of much interest, thinking they will not succeed even if they try; they may have few if any aspirations for the future; they may see antisocial behaviour as a way of keeping in with peers, which is more important than approval from – or respect for – teachers. Some of these young people can be helped by providing some sort of vocational training, but many will not engage even in this. Almost *one in seven* 16–18 year olds in England were not engaged in education, employ-ment or training (NEET) in November 2009. The origins of this malaise usually lie much earlier, for instance in having special educational needs or in the emergence of behaviour problems that are severe enough to lead to suspension or exclusion. These two issues are closely related. For instance:

➤ three-quarters of children who are excluded are identified as having special educational needs
➤ twenty-seven per cent of children with autistic spectrum disorder have been excluded from school
➤ looked-after children are seven times more likely to be excluded than their peers
➤ exclusion rates are as much as 17 times higher than the average for some groups of children identified as having special educational needs.

The report from which these statistics are taken, by the Demos independent think tank, recognises that tackling this sort of disengagement once it has already started is doomed to failure: the roots need to be tackled by a coordinated programme of prevention and early intervention. If these roots are *not* tackled, many of these young people rely on benefits and/or get involved in a variety of criminal activities – both of which cost more than the preventive measures would. Measures that could make a difference include those in the following list; to justify funding, these should be evidence-based and of proven cost-effectiveness, to the extent that available research allows:

➤ better detection and management of ***postnatal depression*** (*see* Chapter 14)
➤ more universal provision and better training of ***health visitors***, who can, for instance, be trained to treat postnatal depression effectively[22] or advise on how to enrich a child's language development[23]
➤ increasing the take-up of ***parenting groups*** (*see* Chapter 13). Unfortunately, parents who need services the most are the least likely to access them. Authori-tative parenting with the following components seems most likely to encourage children to be educationally engaged:
   — providing stability and security in the home environment
   — providing warmth, love and support
   — setting consistent rules (for instance about homework)
   — having positive expectations and aspirations for the child's education.
➤ universal ***preschool provision*** (nursery schooling) that is of *high quality*,[24] which means having:
   — a trained teacher as manager, and a good proportion of trained teachers on the staff
   — a holistic attitude to child development, viewing educational and social development as equally important
   — warm, responsive interactions between staff and children
   — small class sizes and high adult-to-child ratios
   — age-appropriate curricula and stimulating materials in a safe physical setting
   — a language-rich environment

    — high and consistent levels of child participation with a mix of adult-initiated and child initiated interactions – not just free play – so that staff interact with, rather than direct, children in their learning.

➤ like parenting groups, **Sure Start** children's centres have not always, at least in their first few years, been able to attract the parents who most need them, but they have provided an infrastructure within which children and their parents have benefitted in at least some ways, perhaps even more so after the programmes have become well established.[25]

    — Parents find looking after their children less of a struggle.

    — Parents adopt more positive parenting techniques (and show less negative parenting).[26]

    — Parents provide a better home learning environment.

    — Parents are more able to work with relevant services supporting child and family development.

    — Children are given more opportunities at home to learn.

    — Children show more positive social behaviour.

    — Children show more independence and self-regulation.

➤ also needed are earlier detection and more effective remediation of **special educational needs**, particularly literacy, numeracy and communication skills

➤ better **training of teachers** in understanding and managing disruptive behaviour in the classroom

➤ teaching children **personal, emotional and social skills** such as: empathy, self-regulation and how to express emotions other than through behaviour. An example is the Social and Emotional Aspects of Learning (SEAL) programme[27]

➤ provision of interesting and motivating **after-school activities**

➤ dealing effectively with **bullying** (*see* Chapter 22)

➤ **alternatives to exclusion** as a means of dealing with an unruly pupil, such as specialist provision for such pupils within the school (using a learning support or behavioural support unit); or making the provision of education after an exclusion the responsibility of the same school.

Many of these solutions, being educational initiatives, are outside the scope of this book, which takes mainly a problem-focused and health-oriented approach – but they are important examples of a holistic understanding of children's mental health.

SUMMARY

This book is written to support the work of primary mental health workers and others engaged in improving children's mental health and emotional wellbeing – which now means *everybody* who has any contact with children. It is targeted especially at those members of frontline (Tier 1 or universal) services who wish to enhance their skills, whether or not they have access to a primary mental health worker. It would be helpful for anyone who wants to know more about what can be done to help children and young people presenting with problems of living.

REFERENCES

1 Williams R, Richardson G, Kurtz Z, *et al*. The definition, epidemiology and nature of child and adolescent mental health problems and disorders. In: Health Advisory Service. *Child and Adolescent Mental Health Services: together we stand*. London: HMSO; 1995. pp. 15–25.

2 Department for Children, Schools and Families and Department of Health, UK. *Children and young people in mind: the final report of the National CAMHS Review*. London: DCSF and DH; 2008. p. 5. Available at: www.dh.gov.uk/en/Publicationsandstatistics/Publications/PublicationsPolicyAndGuidance/DH_090399 (accessed 20 March 2011).

3 Health Advisory Service, op. cit.

4 Although not necessarily credited, the authors of this report included Peter Hill, Richard Williams, Zarina Kurtz, Peter Wilson and William Parry-Jones.

5 National CAMHS Review, op. cit. p. 17, Box 1.

6 National CAMHS Review, op. cit. p. 61, Section 6.6.

7 National CAMHS Review, op. cit. p. 61, Section 6.6.

8 www.education.gov.uk/childrenandyoungpeople/strategy/integratedworking/caf/a0068957/the-caf-process

9 National CAMHS Review, op. cit. p. 18.

10 National CAMHS Review, op. cit. p. 6.

11 National CAMHS Review, op. cit. p. 37. *Summary of key findings from focus groups and interviews with children, young people, parents and carers, conducted specifically for the Independent CAMHS Review Expert Group* [with some grammatical alterations].

12 www.cwdcouncil.org.uk/common-core

13 Layard R, Dunn J. *A Good Childhood: searching for values in a competitive age*. London: The Children's Society and Penguin Books; 2009.

14 Wilkinson R, Pickett K. *The Spirit Level: why more equal societies almost always do better*. London: Allen Lane; 2009.

15 The United Nations Children's Fund. *Child poverty in perspective: an overview of child well-being in rich countries. A comprehensive assessment of the lives and well-being of children and adolescents in the economically advanced nations*. Report Card 7. Florence, Italy: UNICEF Innocenti Research Centre; 2007. Available at: www.unicef-irc.org/publications/pdf/rc7_eng.pdf (accessed 20 March 2011).

16 Marmot M. *Fair Society, Healthy Lives: strategic review of health inequalities in England post-2010* [Marmot review final report]. London: University College; 2010. Available at: www.marmotreview.org (accessed 28 April 2011).

17 Equality and Human Rights Commission. *How Fair is Britain? Equality, human rights and good relations in 2010*. London: 2010. sec 10.1. Available at: www.equalityhumanrights.com/key-projects/triennial-review/full-report-and-evidence-downloads (accessed 20 March 2011).

18 www.dh.gov.uk/en/Publicationsandstatistics/Publications/PublicationsPolicyAndGuidance/DH_118530

19 Kennedy I. Getting it right for children and young people. Overcoming cultural barriers in the NHS so as to meet their needs. London: Department of Health; 2010. Available at: www.dh.gov.uk/en/Publicationsandstatistics/Publications/PublicationsPolicyAndGuidance/DH_119445 (accessed 20 March 2011).

20 McMillan HL, Wathen CN, Barlow J, *et al*. Interventions to prevent child maltreatment and associated impairment. *Lancet*. 2009; **373:** 250–66.

21 Sodha S, Margo J. *A generation of disengaged children is waiting in the wings* [Ex Curricula]. London: Demos; 2010. Available at: www.demos.co.uk/files/Ex-curricula_-_web.pdf? 1267034385 (accessed 20 March 2011).

22 Morrell CJ, Slade P, Warner R, *et al.* Clinical effectiveness of health visitor training in psychologically informed approaches for depression in postnatal women: pragmatic cluster randomised trial in primary care. *BMJ.* 2009; **338:** a3045.

23 Sutton C, Utting D, Farrington D, editors. *Support from the Start: working with young children and their families to reduce the risks of crime and anti-social behaviour.* London: Department for Education and Skills; 2004. As quoted in Sodha, 2010, op. cit.

24 Sylva K, Melhuish E, Sammons P, *et al. Final Report From the Primary Phase: pre-school, school and family influences on children's development during Key Stage 2.* London: Department for Children, Schools and Families; 2008. As quoted in Sodha, 2010, op. cit.

25 Melhuish E, Belsky J, Leyland AH, *et al.* Effects of fully-established Sure Start Local Programmes on 3-year-old children and their families living in England: a quasi-experimental observational study. *Lancet.* 2008; **372:** 1641–7.

26 Hutchings J, Bywater T, Daley D, *et al.* Parenting intervention in Sure Start services for children at risk of developing conduct disorder: pragmatic randomised controlled trial. *BMJ.* 2007; **334:** 678–82.

27 Department for Children, Schools and Families. *Social and Emotional Aspects of Learning (SEAL): improving behaviour, improving learning.* London: Department for Children, Schools and Families; 2005. Available at: http://nationalstrategies.standards.dcsf.gov.uk/ primary/publications/banda/seal (accessed 20 March 2011).

CHAPTER 2

Preschool

INTRODUCTION

This chapter will focus on the vast number of physiological, cognitive and psycho-social changes that occur during this developmental stage, and on how to engage, assess and work with preschool children and their families. As there are so many changes that occur during this period, we can realistically attempt to give only a brief summary. It will cover from early infancy through toddlerhood up to the age of five years. As attachment is discussed in Chapter 7, this chapter will instead attempt to highlight what could be considered within the normal range of child-hood development, to enable recognition of whether the difficulties that carers describe, or the child's observed behaviour, require further professional attention. Parental anxiety about preschool children is to be expected, whether development is outside the normal range or not.

Comparisons

Comparing oneself to others is an unavoidable part of human behaviour. It is a method we all employ, for instance, to check whether our behaviour is acceptable. Even before conception, some parents-to-be may exchange comparisons as a way of checking that they have what it takes to be a good parent. They may compare themselves with friends, relatives and strangers on factors such as age, health and finances. There is presumably an evolutionary advantage to making comparisons with others – perhaps it increases the likelihood of becoming a successful parent and so propagating genes into the next and subsequent generations. Measuring up to others is also clearly evident in pregnancy: some mothers compare their physical symptoms or the shape of the bump. After the babies are born, compari-sons may continue, with parents sharing stories about the birth, current feeding and sleeping routines and developmental milestones. Although parents may have always swapped tales and learnt from each other in this way, the likelihood of seeking professional advice about small children may have increased. This may be related to a decrease in seeking advice from previous generations of the extended family – which in turn may be because of the increasing geographical dispersion of families, due often to the search for career opportunities. Combined with rapid changes in technology and working patterns, such family fragmentation may have reduced the extent to which wisdom and knowledge are passed down from one generation to the next.

Learning how to parent

If we briefly consider learning theory, we can discern three different ways in which we learn:
➤ modelling
➤ direct experience
➤ following instructions.

Parents may base much of how they parent on how, as children, they experienced being parented (the first bullet point above). This is despite memories under the age of about four to five years not being fully developed, not least because of the importance of language in registering and retrieving memories. It is unlikely, for instance, that we will recall as parents when or how we first learnt as children to string sentences together, to use the toilet independently or to manage developmentally appropriate fears (such as fear of the dark or fear of strangers). Direct experience may be a valuable teacher, but many parents want something more. Instruction from familiar adults – especially grandparents – may be unavailable (or perhaps unwanted). Some parents may have good support networks on which to draw for advice as a substitute for having their own parents readily available, but others less so. All of this has led to an increase in the sales of parenting manuals, reliance on a variety of professionals and the use of the internet as a source of advice (*see* Box 2.1).

BOX 2.1 Case Example

Lucy has had concerns about her son Tom's speech development for some time. Her daughter Abigail learnt to speak from about the age of two years, and has been able to hold a two-way conversation since she was three years old. In contrast, at Tom's third birthday, his maternal grandparents – visiting from Ireland – make comments about his behaviour and language that fuel Lucy's anxiety. Lucy recalls how Tom has been later than Abigail with **all** of his milestones and is still not fully toilet-trained, which Abigail was by her third birthday. Her parents say that their other grandchildren are much more advanced than Tom, so suggest Lucy should take him to the doctor's to get him checked.

Lucy raises her concerns initially with her health visitor at Tom's three-year check. The health visitor asks if Tom's playgroup has ever voiced any concerns: Lucy says they have not, but then realises that she has never asked. The health visitor checks with Lucy how Tom compares to friends or relatives of his age. Lucy explains that they rarely mix with peers except at parties, and most of the extended family live in Ireland – it is her parents' comparison to Tom's cousins that has started her worrying. The health visitor spends some time playing with Tom, using the toy cars he has found in the room. She also asks Tom to look through a storybook with her and talk about the pictures in the book.

The health visitor can find no cause for concern from her assessment but mentions to Lucy that it is good she has mentioned her anxieties about his development.

She encourages Lucy to speak with the playgroup staff to check if they too have any concerns. The health visitor speaks about the differences in development between all children and in particular between boys and girls. With experience of only one other child, it would be difficult for Lucy to appreciate the wide range of normal development. The health visitor directs Lucy to some reading material and suggests she should come back if her concerns continue, or if there **are** any concerns at playgroup.

A developmental perspective

Parents compare their child's development to what they consider 'normal', but no two children ever follow exactly the same course: each child gains skills at her own rate. Children usually gain these skills in a similar sequence; for example, most children will say single words before speaking in sentences. However, it is common for one child to be ahead of another child in one area, such as language, but behind in a different area, such as motor skills. Gender differences may play a part in this, with girls being on average a few months ahead of boys regarding their first motor and speech milestones. What is clear is that developmental milestones vary greatly and can be influenced by a variety of factors. Below is merely a brief guide to 'average' development.

Biological development

The biological changes during infancy and early childhood may be the easiest for parents to appreciate. During the first 18 months there are rapid changes in weight, body proportions, height, skeletal development, muscular development and brain growth. For example, at birth the head is significantly disproportionate to the body, so the baby's muscle tone cannot hold the head up until about four months. Other motor milestones are shown in Table 2.1.

Olfactory (smell) recognition is present at birth, sufficient to enable discrimination of the bay's own mother's milk from another mother's. Together with voice recognition, this complements and encourages the gradually developing ability to recognise familiar adults visually. A newborn has very immature vision and so is

TABLE 2.1 Gross motor developmental milestones

Action	Age
Rolls over	3–5 months
Sits without support	5–8 months
Stands holding on	6–10 months
Walks holding on	9–13 months
Stands alone	11–14 months
Walks alone	11–18 months

attracted to moving objects that have a high contrast, preferring complex patterns such as faces to simpler ones. Between three and six months infants become more able to perceive form, make complex visual discriminations and understand the correspondence between what they see and what they touch. This enables recognition of familiar faces and the dawning of a fear of heights. From six months on, visual perception becomes more adept, with better judgments of size, depth, speed and form.

By the age of two years, most children are relatively strong on their feet. The majority can walk unaided, run, cope with steps and kick a ball. Their fine motor skills are also developing with most able to hold a pencil and draw simple, if unidentifiable, forms on a page. At this age physical development begins to slow a little and children begin to look taller and leaner. Over the next few years there are significant improvements in fine motor control and hand-eye coordination.

By the age of three years children can run fairly proficiently, ride a tricycle, feed themselves, draw a circle, put on their own shoes and pour themselves a drink. By four years most can hop on one foot, dress themselves and draw a recognisable figure. By five years their balance has improved considerably, enabling them to hop, skip, skate and ride a two-wheeled bike – initially perhaps with stabilisers. Their fine-motor control continues to improve, enabling them to fasten buttons, do their own shoelaces and begin to write recognisable letters.

Cognitive development

During early infancy (up to two years) Piaget[1] described infants going through what he termed the '*sensori-motor*' stage of cognitive development in which they begin to develop rudimentary thought. This is a period in which the child learns about the world through interaction with it and the experience of observing consequences. By 8–12 months an infant has developed intentionality, meaning that movements and other actions appear planned. This is demonstrated by the ability to imitate gestures and copy actions. The infant learns to anticipate what will happen next, which can be clearly seen in simple games such as peek-a-boo. By 10–12 months an infant has usually developed object permanence, meaning that she will search for an object that has moved out of her field of view. By 18–24 months early symbolic play has developed alongside simple problem-solving skills. At this age, a toddler is also able to follow simple instructions involving two or even three parts, for instance: 'Please pick up the doll and put it in the toy box'.

Next comes the '*pre operational*' stage of cognitive development, between the ages of two to seven years. During this period, a child's symbolic play and reasoning develops significantly, as language develops. Prior to this age, a child's interaction with the world is immediate and dependent on the objects in close proximity around her. During this stage of development, in contrast, the child begins to be able to carry mental representations from one situation to another. For example, a two year old may observe another child having a temper tantrum in the supermarket and consequently acquiring parental attention. A week later, in a different supermarket, she may herself recreate the exact same behaviour, apparently also with the same aim. The child's play also begins to be more representational, with imaginative use of objects. For example, a child may pretend a cardboard box is a rocket going to the moon, where she meets monsters who eat jelly and ice cream all day. The child can also now make some interesting generalisations, creating categories or rules. She may refer, for instance, to all men over a certain age as 'granddad' (much to the embarrassment of her parents). Another example is that a child who has been scratched by a cat may show indiscriminate fear of all furry four-legged creatures, expecting every one of them to scratch her. As the child's language develops further, adult explanations of rules and concepts may be enough for new learning to take place, although direct experience may still provide a stronger stimulus to remembering.

A key aspect of this stage of development is the tendency for the child to view the world from her own perspective and to have difficulty with recognising another person's point of view. Piaget termed this '*ego-centrism*'. By the age of four years, a child's theory of mind is beginning to develop, and she is better able to judge the thoughts and feelings of others. This is the age that friendships really start to flourish.

At the same time, the child's ability to concentrate, plan and recall information is also developing. For example, in the first year of life, recognition of objects and familiar faces is apparent. By the age of two years, children are usually able to recall interesting events that have occurred in the recent past. By three years, a child's long-term memory has significantly developed, often much to the surprise of her parents when she claims to recall an event from up to a year previously. By the age of four years, a child can be highly imaginative, may ask endless questions and has learnt to generalise. By five years, concentration and attention have improved significantly. Children of this age are able to differentiate between fact and fiction.

Language development

Although infants do not utter their first meaningful words till around the age of one year, there is considerable language development in this period and the following few years. Early crying and babbling quickly begin to take on qualities such as tone, pitch and volume, enabling the child to communicate meaningfully and parents to discriminate the child's needs. Infants from the age of four months begin to recognise turn-taking in language and the power of their verbal communication.

Between 12–18 months, infants begin to say clear, recognisable words. In this early stage, their vocabulary tends to develop by one word at a time; parents may recount the number of words their child can now say. From 18–24 months, children begin to combine words into simple sentences. This early language consists mostly of nouns and verbs, particularly describing objects that are of interest to them.

By the age of two years, comprehension of language has greatly increased and children are beginning to make longer utterances. When a child reaches three years, grammar is also developing: children become able to name relational contrasts such as objects being big or small, long or short, and they are also beginning to use plurality. They show an amazing ability to apply the grammatical rules they have learnt, but (to adult amusement) not always correctly – making neologisms such as: 'sheeps', 'foots', 'brung', 'buyed' or 'thinked'. This demonstrates the ability to learn rules and apply them rather than just repeating language previously heard. Babbling, making up words and rhyming (mummy, yummy, summy, lummy) are common and are presumably a way of developing language skills.

By four years, a child is speaking in complete sentences and uses language as a tool to acquire information – hence the endless questions that parents may struggle to answer patiently. By five years, the child has mastered a great deal of grammar and a sizeable vocabulary, so can speak in a relatively sophisticated manner. But language is not yet fully developed, and continues to be enriched through childhood and adolescence.

Psychosocial development

What a child learns about herself, her relationships and the world around her during early childhood is the foundation from which she subsequently develops socially and personally. Erikson[2] proposed an eight-stage theory of psychosocial development across the lifespan which aims to explain how an individual develops an identity combined with an understanding of the world. He proposed that one of the key elements of psychosocial development is the forming of an individual's 'ego identity'. In other words, how an individual views herself is mainly based on and learnt from her interactions with others. He described how during our lives we pass from one stage to the next (probably with some overlap); three of the stages are in the preschool years.

The first stage is that of '***trust versus mistrust***'. During the first couple of years of life, an infant is learning from her interactions with caregivers whether or not the world is a good, predictable and safe place. Caregivers who are neglectful, inconsistent, rejecting, abusive or emotionally unavailable can lead a child to develop a belief that the world is unsafe and that people are not to be trusted. This is a period when babies and toddlers often show a preference for key caregivers; stranger awareness is evident intermittently from about nine months.

Erikson's second stage he described as '***autonomy versus shame and doubt***', lasting from about 18 months to four years. Sometimes referred to as 'the terrible twos', this period is often regarded by parents as turbulent, due to children attempting to exert more control. Erikson viewed the child during this period as developing her independence and awareness of personal control. Parents who can facilitate in their children the development of a sense of autonomy will lead them also to become more self-confident. Toilet-training is a key milestone during this stage, in which a child is able to experience and demonstrate both personal control and independence. There are other opportunities to involve a child in decision-making, for example about what T-shirt to wear or what piece of fruit to eat, which can all help to facilitate her autonomy and satisfy her need for control. Children who do not experience opportunities to exert control and choice may struggle to make decisions and become too dependent on adults.

The third Eriksonian stage covers the age range of 3½ to five years: he called it *'initiative versus guilt'*. This is the period when children are beginning to enjoy the company of their peers and participating in joint play activities. Erikson envisaged a continuum between (at one end) those children who can experience success at taking the lead and directing play; and (at the other end) those children who feel anxious in group situations, including play. The natural leaders and those who feel comfortable in group situations will learn to enhance their own capabilities and to co-operate more effectively in relationships. Those at the socially-anxious end of the continuum will tend to avoid peer interactions or develop self-doubt or guilt about their capabilities. In practice, many children have elements of both ends of this continuum. Turn-taking can help the child develop some degree of mastery in social situations, thus combining the positive elements of the second and third stages.

ASSESSMENT
Parental factors
Assessing a preschool child should include not only an assessment of the child's development and functioning but also an assessment of any carer's functioning, including the extent to which a carer may enhance the child's resilience or add to the child's vulnerability (probably inadvertently). Some degree of anxiety about the parental role is an inevitable part of parenthood – indeed it may be essential to ensure the child's needs are met. A child's anxiety may however be increased by parental anxiety, insecurity or competitiveness. Postnatal depression may put strains on the mother-child relationship, potentially increasing the child's later insecurity or need to obtain attention. Other causes of parental unavailability include major depressive disorder, a bereavement reaction, obsessive-compulsive disorder, domestic violence or drug and alcohol overuse. If alcohol misuse occurred during pregnancy, there may be a biological adverse impact on the child's development (even without full-blown foetal alcohol syndrome). So the family history should include some enquiry about each parent's mental health and functioning, past and present, and that of any other main caregiver. However, even if one or more of these factors are present, it may not necessarily lead to difficulties or developmental delay in the child.

Prenatal factors
Parental anxiety about a child's development may be influenced even before conception (*see* Box 2.2). The pregnancy may have been very long-awaited and it may have required additional medical intervention. There may have been a loss of previous pregnancies or some difficulty carrying this one. Parents may hold religious or cultural beliefs regarding the rights and wrongs of the pregnancy itself, leading them to question if the child is having difficulties because of this. If asked some open-ended questions about the pregnancy, parents will often volunteer information of relevance. Having a stance of curiosity and interest can be more effective at eliciting relevant information than asking lots of questions.

BOX 2.2 Case Example

Due to her return to work part-time, Judy has enrolled her two-year-old daughter Emily into a local private nursery. It is evident from the introductory days that Emily struggles to separate from her mother. Nursery staff observe Emily clinging onto Judy and becoming very distressed whenever she tries to leave. Judy herself appears to the nursery staff as a very warm, caring parent who is also becoming quite distressed at separating – apparently more in response to her daughter's distress than due to not wanting to leave her daughter. Staff at the nursery reassure Judy that this behaviour is common in the initial few weeks and that she should try not to worry. Unexpectedly, this behaviour continues for some months, so Emily's key worker spends some time with Judy to try to understand Emily and find ways of helping her settle.

Judy shares with her key worker the history of Emily being a long-awaited baby. During the pregnancy, Judy spent two months in hospital due to various medical complications. Previously, Judy lost a baby born at 22 weeks gestation. With problems in both her pregnancies, Judy was understandably anxious about Emily when she was born. Initially, she would not let Emily out of her sight, and was so concerned about germs that she was reluctant even to hold her. By the time Emily was two, Judy was much less anxious. She wonders with her key worker whether she overprotected Emily during her first six months. The key worker attempts to empathise with Judy, saying that her protective behaviour towards Emily is understandable given the history; she also emphasises how well Judy is managing the evidently painful task of leaving Emily in childcare. She gives Judy lots of reassurance about how safe Emily will be in the nursery.

They discuss ways of leaving Emily that could decrease the separation anxiety. They conclude that Emily might react in a different way to her father dropping her off, and the subsequent experiment is a success. Over the next few months, Emily's father is able to bring her to nursery in the morning – separating from him seems to trigger much less distress. Emily eventually seems to accept her time in nursery as part of her routine and Judy is able to take over from her husband for the morning drop-off. Although Emily still has the occasional day of becoming quite distressed, this is much less frequent and shorter-lived than previously. Nursery staff find things to interest and distract Emily from the moment she enters the building: examples include going to look at the nursery's hamster or racing a member of staff to the window so that Emily can wave goodbye to mummy as she gets into her car.

Perinatal factors

In addition to the pregnancy, the experience of labour and birth can for some parents be a factor leading to doubts about their child's development. The occurrence of some medical complication, whether affecting child or mother, can lead one or both parents to believe that the baby must be damaged in some way. A mother may question whether her child spending time in a special care baby unit may adversely affect their early relationship. Parents may worry about the impact on their child of difficulties with breast feeding, post-birth illnesses, infections, immunisations or domestic violence.

Organising the assessment

When a parent seeks help or advice from a professional, it is important to understand clearly what she may be concerned about. Some parents may need a particular sort of help, requiring a pointer in the direction of another professional. Others may be seeking reassurance or advice on facilitating their child's development. (For more on the issue of how to understand who wants what and why, *see* Chapter 3 on Middle Childhood.)

It may be helpful to gather information about a child's development and functioning from a range of sources. This can include:

➤ information direct from either parent
➤ observation of the child
➤ observation of interaction between child and parent
➤ observation of interaction between parents, if you can get to see both
➤ information from any other main carer, such as a grandparent
➤ information from any childcare professionals looking after the child, such as a childminder or those working in a playgroup or nursery
➤ reports from anyone else who has seen the child or family.

If only one source of information is available it can be useful to ask the question: 'If X were here today, what would he say about your concerns?'

Relating to the child

Some professionals may be anxious about attempting to gather information from a young child. This can be for a variety of reasons, but often a major factor may be that they are simply not used to it. For some, there may be a myth that there is a right way and a wrong way to gather information from a preschool child.

There may be concern about upsetting a child or about how to pose questions in an age-appropriate manner. Even the most experienced worker may feel self conscious about the effort needed to get onto the child's wavelength, especially when a parent is watching. However, young children are very forgiving, and the majority of parents are happy to help you and the child understand each other, for instance by interpreting the child's speech or elaborating on the child's answers – much as they would do in other environments. Spending some time merely observing the child initially, whilst interacting with the carer, is likely to be the most facilitative way forward. This can enable the child to see that her carer is comfortable with you, with the result that she will feel less anxious herself.

Asking direct questions to children under three years old is likely to elicit a poor response, if any; attempts to engage in play are likely to be much more successful. It is also important not to tower above a person who is much smaller than you: get down to the child's level, by bending, crouching, sitting on the floor or if necessary getting onto all fours to play. Simple materials such as paper and coloured crayons or felt-tips can keep most children of two years and above somewhat entertained and can then be used as a way of engaging and joining the child. Having some age-appropriate toys available can provide not only a way of relaxing the child but also a means of non-verbal communication.

MANAGEMENT

Support

If it is evident from your assessment that what a parent needs is support, reassurance or advice about her child's development, it is best if possible not to pathologise the child (or the parental concerns!).

Some parents may benefit from a local parent support group. For some a generic group may be sufficient, such as an under-ones' group or a toddler play group; for others, a targeted group may provide more support and information, such as a breast-feeding support group or a single parents' group. Health visitors are usually the best fount of knowledge on what is available locally; a search of the local authority's website may also be helpful.

Care from members of the extended family such as grandparents may also offer an opportunity for the child to develop psychosocial skills whilst giving tired parents a chance to recharge their batteries.

Knowledge

Your assessment may have highlighted a lack of knowledge in a particular area. Helping the parent access accurate up-to-date information, and providing sensitive support and guidance, may be all that is required. This may be through discussion, or suggested reading, or suggested websites, or a combination. Given the wealth of information available on parenting, some guidance will be needed as to which websites and books are likely to be most helpful (*see* resources below). In some areas there are book prescribing schemes, sometimes called bibliotherapy, that ensure ample supplies of appropriate books are available at relevant clinics or public libraries.

Relationship with professionals

Whatever a parent's main question or concern, it is very important that she feels heard and taken seriously. This contact early in the child's life with any professional can have a lasting influence on how a parent seeks help for her child in the future – much like the impact of a child's early experience of school. If it is experienced as positive and non-blaming, parents are more likely to be open in sharing information and feelings, and receptive to thinking about different ways of doing things.

Parents, carers and workers in regular contact with children and their parents can enhance a child's development in many different ways.

Exercise

It is important with any child to encourage movement from an early age and give plenty of opportunity for exercise. This not only helps to develop muscle tone, co-ordination and balance but can also help to expend excess energy. Unspent energy can contribute to behavioural difficulties. A child who learns new physical skills such as kicking a ball, catching a balloon or riding a bicycle will experience mastery and an increase in self-confidence. Regular activity with others can also be an opportunity for the child to develop social skills and the parent to mix with other parents. Examples include: baby gym, adventure playgrounds, swimming pools or dancing classes.

Diet

Encouraging healthy eating from an early age can also aid physical development. Some parents may benefit from straightforward information about how to provide a balanced diet. Eating together as a family at least once a day can also help to develop good eating habits and facilitate communication between family members, especially if the television is turned off for the duration of the meal (*see also* Chapter 44 on Diet and Exercise).

Cognitive development

An infant's cognitive development can be encouraged by facilitating the safe exploration of the environment and objects around her. Straightforward advice on child-proofing the home environment can help, for instance by decreasing parental anxiety and by allowing the child a freer rein to explore. Providing a wide range of play activities and environments to explore helps to stimulate all the senses. There should be times for both indoor and outdoor play; both quiet, calm play and noisy rough-and-tumble play. There should be opportunities to explore new textures, smells and tastes. Rotating the selection of toys that are most immediately available can decrease the likelihood of boredom, particularly in very young children, who show a preference for novel stimuli. The purchase of toys at different times of the year, such as birthdays or Christmas, can be a way of ensuring that at least some toys are age-appropriate. Children whose birthday falls very close to Christmas should perhaps have half-birthdays!

Concerns about cognitive development may come to the fore once a child is within a nursery or school setting, through observation by experienced staff. If their concerns match parental worries, then some action is warranted. Initially, it may be sufficient to explore ways of enhancing developmental progress and monitor closely. In all preschool and school settings, access to special educational needs support is available, providing ideas on how best to promote a child's development. If cognitive development is clearly delayed, and does not improve with combined parental and professional attention, then referral may be indicated, either to a community paediatrician or an educational psychologist.

Language development

Language development can be greatly advanced at all ages by any adult in appreciable contact with the child taking the time to talk with her. Regular reading to the child (by an adult or older child) can expose her to the sounds and rhythms of language, increase her vocabulary, stimulate her imagination and provide some positive one-to-one time. Mealtimes, as noted above, can be an opportunity to develop everyone's conversation skills. Some parents may be particularly anxious about language development; this may be related to the huge variation in language skills between children of the same age. In some families, there seems to be a strong family history of expressive language delay (without any long-term consequences). Many children experience transient pronunciation difficulties or stuttered speech, all of which can be part of normal language development. There can be many other causes for delay in speech or language. If parents and professionals at nursery or school are concerned, referral to a speech and language therapist should be considered.

Psychosocial development

A child's capacity for social exploration can be supported by carers helping her to feel as safe and secure as possible. This is particularly important in the first two years of life when the child is developing her beliefs about safety and trust. In whatever setting, whether it is at home, with grandparents, at nursery or at school, having a clear structure, a predictable routine and consistent rules can help children feel contained and secure, and experience the world as a predictable place. Through experiencing clear limits and boundaries, the child can also begin to learn ways of developing self-control.

From an early age, and particularly from the age of two years onwards, contact with other children can greatly facilitate a child's social development. This need not be in a formal, structured way such as within a nursery setting or parent toddler group – informal contact may also help. Examples include: meeting up with parents who have similar-aged children, going to a playground or indoor children's play area, or visiting relatives. Exposure to peers or cousins (in addition to her own siblings) can enhance a child's skills in co-operative play such as turn-taking and sharing. From three years onwards, social opportunities can also enhance her self-confidence and independence.

REFERRAL

If the assessment indicates that a carer is having particular difficulty promoting a child's development, then it may be worth considering what support, in addition to your own, may be helpful and accessible. Further support may be given by advising a parent to access help that is directly for herself – for example, for her own mental health problem or substance misuse – or looking at whether additional practical support may be needed. Support may come in a variety of forms.

If you think that further assessment is necessary, then refer to the appropriate professional: for example, a community paediatrician, a speech and language therapist or a dietician. Assessment, management and referral in relation to specific concerns is covered in further detail in other chapters of this book.

BOX 2.3 Case Example

Satwinder is two-and-a-half years old when he starts at nursery. At first, he seems very shy, but he quickly becomes able to separate from his mother. Two months after he starts, he seems to have got used to interacting with the other children, but he does not seem able to follow instructions, and begins to show signs of frustration when asked to share toys. The nursery school staff tell his mother, Shruthi, that they cannot understand why he is becoming so aggressive, as he seemed such a nice quiet boy to start with.

Shruthi mentions this to her health visitor at the three-year check. Amongst other questions, the health visitor asks whether Shruthi has any concerns about Satwinder's hearing. Shruthi says initially that she hasn't noticed much, but then remembers that he had a bad cold six weeks ago: she realises during this conversation that, since then, she has had to make sure he is looking at her before he will do what she tells him – she assumed this was just his age. The health visitor is not able to test Satwinder's hearing herself, but she refers him to the community paediatrician who specialises in audiological testing.

Satwinder is found to have glue ear, with a 20-decibel loss on the left and a 30 decibel loss on the right – enough to make him struggle to hear in noisy rooms. As he has recently had a cold, this is not given active treatment at first, but is merely reviewed again after six weeks. Unfortunately, it remains just as bad, so Satwinder is referred to an ear, nose and throat surgeon for grommets. By the end of the following term, Satwinder's hearing is back to normal, and he is getting on very well with the staff and pupils of the nursery school.

BOX 2.4 Practice Points for the assessment and management of preschool children

Expect every parent to have some anxiety about her child's development.

Remember that children develop at different rates, so there is huge variation in the age at which different children reach the same developmental milestone.

Listen to what the carer is most concerned about and attempt to address that.

The family's health visitor may have a great deal of knowledge about the child, family and wider network that can be accessed to provide the support or help that is needed.

If appropriate, gather as much information as you can about a child's development from a variety of sources.

Encourage contact with other parents as a source of comparative information and advice swapping.

Encourage parents to facilitate the child's contact with peers to enhance the development of social skills.

TABLE 2.2 Alarm Bells in the assessment of preschool children

Parental issues	Child issues
Poor parental mental health	Falling off height and weight centiles
Parental substance misuse	Concern about hearing
Domestic violence	Failure to develop speech
Neglect or other forms of abuse	Extreme anxiety in the child in a range of situations
	Marked difficulty separating from a parent
	No interest in peers from the age of two years

RESOURCES
Books for children on developmental challenges
- Moser A, Melton M. *Don't Rant & Rave on Wednesdays! The children's anger-control book.* Kansas City: Landmark Editions Inc; 1994.
  This book describes common and inappropriate behaviours and suggests ways to control anger and express feelings.
- Ross T. *Little Princess – I Want My Potty.* London: HarperCollins Children's Books; 2006.
  A little princess, tired of nappies, learns to use the potty, although it is not always easy.
- Weiner M, Neimark J, Adinolfi J. *I Want Your Moo: a story for children about self-esteem.* Washington DC: Magination Press (American Psychiatric Association); 2009.
  A turkey despises the sound of her own 'gobble-gobble' and would like to be more like her friend the cow.

Books for parents on child development and how to improve it
- Manolson A. *It Takes Two To Talk: a parent's guide to helping children communicate.* Ontario: The Hanen Centre; 1985.
  Guide for parents to learn how to encourage a child to communicate. It explains different ways to establish a special bond between parent and child.
- Murray L, Andrews L. *The Social Baby: understanding babies' communication from birth.* Richmond: CP Publishing; 2005.
  Looks at ways of helping to promote and develop a child's relationships during the first year.
- Parker J, Stimpson J, Rowe D. *Raising Happy Children: what every child needs their parents to know – from 0 to 11 years.* London: Mobius; 2004.
  This book helps parents think about a variety of issues without getting bogged down in diagnostic labels.
- Schaefer CE, DiGeronimo TF. *Ages and Stages: a parent's guide to normal childhood development.* Chichester: Jossey Bass (Wiley); 2000.
  Describes childhood development from birth to 10 years; also available in audio format.
- Sheridan M, Sharma A, Cockerell H. *From Birth to Five Years: children's developmental progress.* 3rd ed. London: Routledge; 2007.
  The latest edition of this classic text sets out each stage of normal development in young children.
- Welford H. *Successful Potty Training.* London: Thorsons (for the National Childbirth Trust); 2002.
  This is a mine of useful information and handy tips.

Books for professionals

- Lindon J. *Understanding Child Development: linking theory and practice.* London: Hodder Education; 2005.
- Schaffer HR. *Introducing Child Psychology.* Chichester: John Wiley and Sons; 2003.

Websites

- Homestart: www.home-start.org.uk
  This is a network of trained parent volunteers who provide support to families with at least one child under five years to build their confidence and ability to cope.
- Netmums: www.netmums.com
  Netmums is a unique local network for mums with a wealth of information and advice on being a mum or dad in your home town.
- Parentline: www.parentlineplus.org.uk
  This site offers a free 24/7 parents helpline and web information providing parenting advice and parental guidance on a wide range of parenting issues.
- Royal College of Psychiatrists: www.rcpsych.ac.uk
  The Royal College of Psychiatrists' website contains information for the public about a range of issues to do with children and young people including lists of books for parents and carers and children.
- Surestart: www.education.gov.uk/childrenandyoungpeople/earlylearningandchildcare/surestart
  Sure Start is the government's programme to deliver the best start in life for every child by bringing together early education, childcare, health and family support.

REFERENCES

1 Piaget J. Piaget's theory. In: Mussen PH, editor. *Carmichael's Manual of Child Psychology (Volume 1).* New York, NY: Wiley; 1970. pp. 703–32.
2 Erikson EH. Eight ages of man. *International Journal of Psychiatry.* 1966; **2**: 281–300.

CHAPTER 3

Middle childhood

INTRODUCTION

'Middle childhood' refers to the stage of growth and development between the ages of five and 12 years, or until the onset of adolescence. This chapter describes the vast range of developmental changes that occur during this period and how to engage, assess and work with these children and their families.

During this stage, children continue to grow and develop physically, cognitively, socially and emotionally. Because so much of child development happens in the early years and in adolescence, there is a myth that 'nothing much happens' in the gap between. We hope this chapter disproves this myth, although it is true that the rate of change is slower than in the preschool years. A number of psychological theories describe these changes from different perspectives. In Freud's psychoanalytic theory of child development, the term '*latency period*' implies not only that there is less psychosexual development than in the preschool and adolescent years, but also that various energies are being held in reserve ('latent'). The child's observable energies are focused on physical activity and socially accepted or expected activity (such as schoolwork, after-school clubs or play). Other models focus more on the cognitive changes that occur (changes in the child's way of thinking) and refer to middle childhood as the beginning of the '*age of reason*',[1] when children become capable of logical thinking, reasoning and more complex problem-solving.

In addition, the child experiences a number of *social changes* as he enters school: he is given increasing responsibility for his behaviour and how he presents himself in public; he is increasingly influenced by experiences at school and new friends. Together with the home environment, these can shape his sense of identity and self-worth. Adverse experiences at this stage may predispose to the later development of a mental health problem.

From the child's perspective, a combination of significant life events may occur during this period. *Starting school* may be something he finds easy if he has had positive preschool experiences and is of an easy temperament. In contrast, if the child has not had much preschool social experience, is by nature shy, or has an anxious attachment to his mother, he may find adjustment to school relatively traumatic – as may his mother. The parental background (of being parented and being schooled as a child) may influence the child's developing relationship with school, in ways such as the following.

➤ Having had good relationships with teachers as a pupil, she may find it easy to work cooperatively with school staff now.

➤ Having clashed with authority as a child, she may find it difficult to take the side of the teachers when her child clashes with their authority.

➤ Waiting to see a special needs teacher or head teacher may remind her of how she was treated as a naughty child when she was at school.

➤ Having succeeded academically as a child, she may have higher expectations of her own children to succeed.

➤ Having struggled academically as a child, she may have lower expectations of her own children, and possibly even feel threatened when they do too well.

➤ Having been bullied at school she may become very distressed and not know how to react if her own child is bullied.

Other life events that the child may experience at this stage include the ***parent returning to work*** (if not before). This may produce benefits for the family financially and widen the parent's social support network, but can generate difficulties if the parent finds this tiring or stressful or has problems with childcare, and may also lead to the child having less adult quality time with his parent(s). Some type of ***loss*** may be experienced, such as the loss of a pet or the death of a grandparent (*see* Chapter 10 on Death, Dying and Bereavement *and* Chapter 37 on Adjustment Disorder and Post-Traumatic Stress Disorder). Moving house leading to a ***change of school*** or the transition from primary to secondary school or middle to high school are significant events in children's lives. It is easy to underestimate the impact of such changes on the child. The impact may be ameliorated or exacerbated by factors such as: the characteristics of each school, the ability of the child to make new friends, the reasons for the move, and the support provided by the home environment.

During this stage, children may strive for ***acceptance*** and try to conform with peers at school and siblings at home. Not feeling accepted can fuel anxiety or lower self-esteem. Positive peer influences may have as dramatic an effect in bolstering mental health as bullying can in impairing it. Parents may fulfil a vital role by encouraging the positive aspects of peer and sibling relationships, for instance by arranging joint activities or other social opportunities.

From a ***professional*** perspective, working with children in this age range can be very rewarding: they are more articulate than preschoolers and less self-conscious than adolescents. Naturally, it is important to adjust what you say and how you say it to the developmental age of the child. Although some children may be mistrustful of adults, due for instance to abuse or domestic violence, many may accept whatever help you have to offer in a genuine, unquestioning way. Ask the majority of seven year olds a simple question about their life and you will more often than not receive an honest, uncensored answer. This stage of childhood also offers opportunities for change or prevention before any difficulties have become too entrenched.

A DEVELOPMENTAL PERSPECTIVE

Knowledge of the usual sequence and timing of a child's emerging abilities is helpful in understanding the child's difficulties. As at any other age, there is a large amount of variation between individuals and no clear cut-offs between 'normal' and 'abnormal'. Instead, it is better to think about how the child is doing in the three main areas of development: biological, cognitive and psychosocial.

Biological development

Growth during middle childhood is slower than during the preschool period and accelerates again in puberty (hence the aptness of the term 'latency'). The timing of the beginning of the growth spurt can vary greatly: in girls, it can start as young as eight years; in boys, it can be delayed until 15 years. So same-aged peers may differ greatly in height, weight and stage of pubertal development. These differences are mainly genetic, but growth can be impaired by nutritional inadequacy, chronic illness or persistent neglect.

BOX 3.1 Case Example

Rajiv is emotionally abused and neglected by his natural parents, so is put in foster care at the age of six years. Growth records show that he has grown only 5 cm in height since he was last measured at the age of three years, and has fallen from the 75th to the 9th centile. In his first two years in foster care, he grows 17 cm, and catches up in growth to the 50th centile.

Loss of the first **teeth** (baby teeth) begins around the age of six or seven years beginning with the front teeth, leading to a period with gap-toothed smiles. Such is the emotional impact of this experience for some children that as adults they may vividly recall memories of losing particular teeth. The back teeth are lost later, usually around the age of 10–12 years. By early adolescence, most children have acquired all of their adult teeth apart from the 'wisdom' molars at the back.

Children's **gross motor skills** continue to develop during middle childhood, as their skeletal and muscular systems develop alongside maturation of the central nervous system (*see* Chapter 34 on Motor Development). Speed and agility improves, and children acquire new skills (if given appropriate opportunities) such as cycle riding, dancing or skateboarding. Due perhaps to their greater muscle mass, boys tend to outperform girls in gross-motor skills. In contrast, girls tend to outperform boys in the development of *fine motor skills*. Most five to six year olds can draw simple shapes and letters, and are able to use a knife and fork, albeit a little clumsily still at times. Gradually, most children become able to perform more tasks requiring these skills, such as fastening buttons, tying shoelaces, writing legibly and learning to play a musical instrument.

During middle childhood, children become increasingly aware of their own bodies and develop greater self-control. As concentration and stamina increase, time spent performing or practising certain tasks can greatly influence *specific abilities*. For example, the majority of Olympic athletes, professional sportsmen or musicians have trained and developed their skills during this stage.

Cognitive development

A child's *cognitive skills* continue to develop throughout middle childhood, with improvements in language, concentration, memory and problem-solving.

These are facilitated both by formal education and by less formal opportunities to play imaginatively and to indulge in *natural curiosity* about the world, which should be encouraged as much as possible and facilitated through hands-on experience.

By the age of five to six years, the child becomes less egocentric and more capable of seeing and appreciating another person's point of view (*empathy*). This continues to develop as a child learns more about other people and their behaviour.

Between the ages seven to 11 years, Piaget described children entering into the *concrete operational stage* of development,[2] where fantasy or make-believe thinking gives way to more logical thought and reasoning and the development of certain cognitive skills. Piaget named this stage as 'concrete', meaning that children of this age apply their thinking to objects, situations and events that are real in the present or remembered from the past. More abstract or hypothetical reasoning is not developed until adolescence. The child becomes capable of 'mental operations' or logical, systematic thinking about how one thing relates to another, which follows the following four rules.

➤ *Identity*: the properties of an object remain the same; for instance, a pot of red paint will always remain red paint unless another coloured paint is added.

➤ *Compensation*: one action can cause a change in another; for instance, a ball of blue play-dough squashed with the palm of your hand remains the same blue play-dough but becomes a different shape caused by the person's action.

➤ *Reversibility*: this describes the ability to work backwards through the stages that have occurred; for instance, the toy figures just moved clumsily by a younger sibling can be moved back to where they were before.

➤ *Conservation*: this involves the ability to recognise that the properties of an object, such as its height, weight, volume or area, may not change even when its appearance is altered in some way. An example that is easy to visualise involves pouring liquid from a short, wide container to a tall thin cylinder; the weight and volume of the liquid remain the same, although the height increases and it looks a very different shape.

A child is more likely to understand such concepts and develop this way of thinking by practical examples and exploration that enable him to see and find out for himself (rather than merely talking about them). Parents and teachers should build on the child's natural curiosity and encourage the child to carry out simple experiments at school and home: 'Let's see what happens if we tip this water from this tall thin glass into this short fat one'.

Psychosocial development

During middle childhood, the child becomes more aware of his own competence in a number of areas, including social relationships and academic achievements. Erikson described this as the middle of seven stages in his theory of child development: *'**industry versus inferiority**'.*[3] A child whose efforts to develop skills are positively encouraged and rewarded will begin to feel industrious and confident. In contrast, a child whose prior psychosocial development has been unsuccessful, who is inadequately encouraged, or whose opportunities are in some way restricted will begin to feel inferior to his peers. Such a child may begin to doubt his abilities and may not reach his full potential in social relationships or academic achievement. Success in Erikson's three previous stages (*see* Chapter 2 on Preschool) involves the development of trust, autonomy and initiative, all of which will enhance the child's confidence to try new things, help him become industrious and increase the likelihood of his receiving positive feedback.

In middle childhood, while the influence of the family remains strong, the effects of other **social relationships** become increasingly important, for example with school friends and significant adults such as teachers or activity group leaders. A child's developing social competence during this period is the foundation stone of subsequent relationships in adolescence and adulthood, so it is important to pursue any opportunity for promoting these relationships, for instance through after-school clubs, weekend sports clubs or other group activities. Social acceptance becomes increasingly important: most children (even those with developmental difficulties such as autistic spectrum disorders) want very much to be part of a group, although some are choosier than others about which groups to join. From an evolutionary perspective, survival chances may increase with group membership, so there is intrinsic pressure towards achieving group acceptance. As they get older, most children want to be with others of their own age. Being accepted by peers involves:

➤ understanding the unspoken rules and cultural or social norms that are taken for granted by group members
➤ being able to adjust to different situations and follow others' behaviour
➤ having the same interests and preferences.

The experience of acceptance or rejection by peers can greatly influence a child's view of himself as socially competent. Having a best friend, being accepted into social groups or being invited to friends' birthday parties can enhance self-esteem and social confidence. In contrast, repeated negative experiences such as ostracism by groups, name-calling or other bullying may lead to low self-esteem, social anxiety or school refusal.

As well as wanting to be accepted by others of a similar age, pre-adolescent children are keen to **conform to the expectations of significant adults**, including not only parents and teachers but also youth workers, religious leaders and other group organisers. The child's relationship with a significant adult of this sort may have a big impact on his current emotional life and his future relationships (*see* Case Example in Box 3.2). Adults who are encouraging, calm and consistent will empower the child to become self-confident and well-motivated.

BOX 3.2 Case Example

At the age of seven years, Simon's mother takes him repeatedly to his general practitioner with stomach aches and headaches, which lead to his missing a lot of school. The results of the general practitioner's physical examinations are normal, as are routine blood tests and an abdominal ultrasound. His head teacher's concern about this leads to a home visit from the educational welfare officer. Simon's mother says that she has wondered if there might be something bothering Simon at school, as she has noticed that Simon is well enough to play with friends after school and never misses his football practice on a Saturday morning.

Simon's mother tells the educational welfare officer that Simon has been struggling recently to keep up with his school work; he has always been a sensitive child, prone to be anxious and reserved. Simon tells the educational welfare officer that his previous class teacher was 'scary' and 'too strict'; he has been worried that his new class teacher will be the same. He has not told his parents this: they are very surprised. The educational welfare officer liaises with Simon's head teacher and class teacher: the class teacher is aware that she has been increasingly hard on Simon recently – because he has not been keeping up with his class work. Simon has appeared increasingly distractible and unfocused.

After a meeting in school between the educational welfare officer, Simon's parents, his class teacher and his head teacher, it is agreed that Simon will have some additional literacy support. The class teacher subsequently apologises to Simon in the presence of his parents, explaining that she did not mean to make him feel scared, but has merely been concerned about his not doing the work. She thanks him for explaining the problem to everyone and says she will try to make the classroom a happier place for him. She asks if he can try to let her know in future if he is struggling with anything. Simon comes up with the creative idea that he should write anything he is worried about down in his jotter book for his teacher and parents to read; everyone thinks this an excellent plan.

Simon still has some tummy aches and headaches, but his mother insists he should go to school regardless, and both parents encourage him to share with them each day after school what he has achieved and what he has found difficult. So his school attendance improves, as does his class work, with some additional special needs input. Simon also becomes less anxious about his class teacher: the more time he spends with her, the more he begins to like and trust her.

It is important to continue to have at least one positive ***parent-child relationship*** during this period. Attachment theory sees this relationship as the cornerstone (secure base) from which the child develops the confidence to explore other relationships – with both adults and children (*see* Chapter 7 on Attachment Theory and Looked-After Children). Such a relationship can provide the unconditional love and support that the child continues to need. It can also be an important protective factor and act as a buffer if negative experiences or stressful events occur.

The child can use this person to help him make sense of and cope with what has happened.

By the age of seven to eight years most children have developed a capacity to **verbalise thoughts and feelings**. Although the difference is far greater in adolescence, this may already be easier for girls than boys. Some boys learn that 'boys don't cry' or learn by example from other boys or from significant adults that:

➤ it may be better to pretend you don't have feelings
➤ you don't talk about these feelings
➤ the way to express feelings is in the form of behaviour.

As a result of this difference, many boys in middle childhood (and some girls) have difficulty recognising their own feelings and finding words for them. Emotions such as upset, anger or fear may find expression in a variety of behaviours, which may bear little obvious relationship to the underlying emotions. This is known as **externalising**: directing feelings and problems outwards. The opposite coping style is **internalising**: expressing problems or feelings inwards, leading to the development of anxiety, depression or self-harm. It may be as difficult for a child mental health professional as it can be for parents to decipher these hidden feelings, which may be obscured by the impact of their behavioural expression. Although this two-fold distinction may at times appear to be an oversimplification, it can be very useful in understanding what is going on for the child (*see* Case Examples in Boxes 3.3 and 3.4).

BOX 3.3 Case Example

> Francis, aged eight years, is being bullied at school but is too frightened to tell anyone. Instead, he starts screaming at both his parents at home and refusing to do what they tell him. The best way to keep his behaviour manageable at home seems to be to allow him to play motor-racing games on his console.

BOX 3.4 Case Example

> Frances, aged eight years, is being bullied at school but is too frightened to tell anyone. Instead, she becomes very withdrawn in the classroom, is reluctant to see her friends outside school, and spends much of her time at home playing with her doll's house.

In most boys and girls, **awareness of feelings** develops progressively with age, including:

➤ being able to find words to convey to others internal states of mind
➤ differentiating between a variety of emotions
➤ empathy (intuiting others' feelings)

➤ recognising the influence of one's own behaviour on others' thoughts and feelings
➤ considering more than one perspective at a time.

Development of these skills depends on the child having developed 'theory of mind', meaning awareness that other people have different thoughts and feelings from his own. Children on the autistic spectrum have difficulties with this (*see* Chapter 32).

These skills improve the child's chances of social success, due to an increase in sensitive responding to others. Parents or other involved adults (such as a grandparent, a teaching assistant or a youth worker) can help with the development of these skills by encouraging the child to recognise when he is sad or angry or something else, talking about how he feels, problem-solving about what to do when he feels like that and watching out for others' feelings and reactions.

CHANGES IN SOCIETY THAT AFFECT CHILDREN

Children nowadays are growing up in a world that is rapidly changing and very different from the one in which their parents grew up.[4] **Technology** that makes the world so different includes the Internet, games consoles and a variety of other screen-based activities designed to grab attention (such as high-definition television on large screens, DVDs and mobile phones – plus gadgets likely to be freshly marketed between the writing and publishing of this book!). Children spend an average of at least three hours per week using a computer, and an average of at least 16 hours per week watching television or involved with other electronic media.[5] Such technological innovations have not only changed the way adults work but also the way children play and relate to others. Concerns about children's use of the Internet and video games include:
➤ whether this is linked to violent behaviour
➤ the excessive use of these technologies at the expense of other activities and family interaction
➤ possible harmful contacts made online
➤ cyberbullying.

A child's individual background, age and stage of brain development (especially the frontal cortex) influence how he is affected by and responds to these experiences. With maturation of the frontal cortex, the child is able to take greater responsibility for his own behaviour and evaluate risks better.

Research has shown that people behave differently online to the way they behave in the real world:[6] they may develop two different moral codes for the two arenas. This is potentially more complex for a child who is still trying to establish the social rules of the offline world and who may lack the critical skills necessary to evaluate incoming information and to make decisions about how best to keep himself safe.

Regarding **Internet safety,** parents have a key role to play in managing children's access to potentially inappropriate and unsafe material – especially by setting up parental control software properly. Children need to learn what they can do to keep themselves safe – for instance, by not giving contact details online. Promoting a child's resilience to materials and situations he encounters should be encouraged by allowing him to talk openly about what he is doing. Schools, as well as other services for children and families all have a role to play in equipping parents and their children to stay safe online. This work should increasingly be supported by the UK Council for Child Internet Safety.[7,8]

Console games are popular with many children; whilst very few are genuinely addicted to them, children who devote many of their non-school hours to playing with such stimulating software may miss out on opportunities for other forms of development and socialisation. On the other hand, a new form of socialisation becomes possible:

> 'One of the reasons I enjoy playing video games online is that I can interact with people from all over the world and make friends. Most online games have groups of players working together to complete objectives, which can improve team and leadership skills, or just for socialising while playing the game. Some of my best friends are online ones.'[9]

The child's context and what he brings to the games is important.
➤ Can he distinguish fantasy from reality?
➤ How does he respond to the arousal some games generate?
➤ What is he learning from these games – does he do things outside the game that are modelled on what happens inside the game?

The correlation between ***aggressive behaviour*** and watching violence on television is high, but it is higher still with playing violent console games: there is a plethora of evidence that the relationship is at least partly causal.[10] This effect might be less if parents obeyed the age-restrictions recommended on the cover of the game; it seems that parents are more likely to pay attention to the ratings of films than of games, perhaps through less parental understanding of the alternate world these games contain:[11] many parents feel insufficiently skilled even to *try* the games. Other factors are also important and are likely to mediate the impact of the television and the console, including:
➤ membership in an antisocial gang
➤ the relationships between the child and each parent (or the absence of a parent)
➤ being male
➤ having an antisocial parent
➤ having a low intelligence quotient
➤ having experienced parental separation (*see* Chapter 9 on Separation, Divorce and Reconstituted Families)
➤ poverty
➤ parental substance misuse
➤ child substance misuse.

Children are increasingly influenced by various **media**, ranging from magazines and television advertisements to pornographic images accessible via the Internet or via mobile phones. Images of young girls wearing make-up and adult-style clothes have led to concerns about the inappropriate sexualisation of children.[12] Sexualised images and messages may affect the development of children and influence cultural norms.

➤ Girls may come to value their appearance and accept their treatment as objects of desire.
➤ Boys may want to be muscular and macho rather than sensitive and emotionally intelligent.
➤ Friendly relationships between boys and girls may be polluted by premature sexualisation.
➤ Sexuality may come to be linked with violence, for instance through the increasing exposure of children to pornography.
➤ Images of super-thin models portrayed as heroines to be emulated may contribute in part to concerns about body image (*see* Chapter 28 on Eating Disorders).

ASSESSMENT

As at any age, to understand the child's problem, it is necessary to consider:
➤ the child's development
➤ the child's functioning at home, in school and with friends
➤ parental functioning
➤ protective and risk factors – those factors contributing to the development and maintenance of the problem (*see* Chapter 6 on Resilience and Risk).

How to go about an assessment

First, establish what the **presenting problem** is. What is meant by words such as 'behaviour' or 'attitude'? Ask for a specific example. Find out the following.
➤ Who sees it as a problem?
➤ Who has asked for help?
➤ What help does she expect?
➤ Why has she asked now?
➤ How long has she been concerned?
➤ What has been tried already?

Sometimes, parents simply want to know whether the child's behaviour or experiences are something to be concerned about or not: there may not be a close family member or friend with childcare experience from whom they can obtain guidance. Once you have clarified who is worried about what, you can move on to other areas.

Take a **developmental history**.
➤ How was the pregnancy?
➤ What was the labour and birth like (including birth weight, gestational age and any need for paediatric intervention)?

➤ What were the temperamental characteristics in the first year regarding feeding, sleeping and crying?

➤ When did milestones occur in walking, speech and language?

➤ How was nursery school? How did the child separate? How did he relate to other children? Did the staff have any comments or concerns?

➤ Have there been any significant stresses, changes or losses in the child's life so far? This could include parental separation, moving house, domestic violence, maternal depression, parental substance misuse, death of a grandparent and many other examples.

➤ Review the medical history. Any medical condition, particularly a chronic one, can affect a child's mental health, and lead to a presentation with behavioural or emotional difficulties. Ask whether there is any paediatric involvement.

A brief *family history* is also important. This does not need to include details of every relative, but it is helpful to know who is living at home, some details about each parent (such as age and occupation), plus how much contact the child has with any grandparents, other significant adults or an absent parent. Ask about any stresses, changes or losses affecting the main caregiver, and what support is available to her, for instance from the extended family or from friends. (*See also* Chapter 8 on Family Issues.)

Other areas to consider exploring, if appropriate, include the following.

➤ What is the child's daily pattern of *diet and exercise*? Could this be relevant to the presenting complaint? (*See* Chapter 44 on Diet and Exercise.)

➤ What is the family's coping style? How have the child and parents responded to change or adversity in the past? You could ask, for instance, about the transition to full-time school. What are their strengths and *protective factors*? Highlighting strengths and successes can help families feel empowered and optimistic, and contribute to building a therapeutic engagement.

➤ What is the *impact* of the presenting problem on each family member? How has it changed things, and what has it changed? Who has found it easiest or most difficult to deal with? How stressful has it been? How does one family member know how stressed another is? Who has supported whom?

➤ What are the family *beliefs or attitudes* to the problem? For instance, a belief that the problem is biological or hereditary can either lead families to feel powerless to effect change or help them to accept that the problem is not their fault, so enabling them to generate solutions. Other beliefs may lead to parents blaming the child or feeling responsible themselves, which can at times be paralysing and inhibit change.

➤ What *solutions* have family members already found to the presenting problem? When have there been exceptions to the general routine in the way the problem occurs? For example, have there been times when the child has accepted being told he can't have something *without* having a tantrum? What enabled this exception? What made things work all right then? Who did what differently? This emphasis on solutions and exceptions can help steer the therapeutic conversation in a positive direction and empower family members to realise they have the capacity to solve things themselves, without waiting for the professional to do it for them.

➤ Asking a parent about **_her own experiences as a child_** can help explain what makes some stages or problems more difficult than others. For example, in relation to bullying (*see* Chapter 22): a parent who has been through similar experiences as a child and found ways of coping is more likely to be able to help her children develop successful strategies than a parent who suffered from victimisation as a child without finding a way out.

Time constraints will limit the choice of which of these avenues to pursue, which will also depend upon the nature and severity of the presenting problem and the environments in which it is most apparent. Gathering such information can be done in a variety of ways – using a **_variety of sources_** that may add valuable complementary information from different viewpoints.

Conversations can be held with the child, parent(s) and siblings in various combinations, including:

➤ all together
➤ parent(s) alone
➤ child alone (*see* below)
➤ child and parents without siblings
➤ child and siblings without parents.

Observations can be made of:

➤ the child's interactions with other family members
➤ the child in the professional's office or any other setting in which you are meeting him or her
➤ the child at home
➤ the child at school
➤ the parents' interactions with each other.

Other sources of information about the child (and family) to consider are:

➤ staff at the child's school
➤ other family members, such as a grandparent
➤ other involved professionals, such as the general practitioner, social worker, speech and language therapist, educational psychologist, social inclusion pupil support worker or educational welfare officer (*see* Figure 1.1 in Chapter 1 on context).

Once all this information is available, it can be summarised in the form of a **_grid_** using four types of causal factors on one axis (**predisposing, precipitating, perpetuating and protective**) and three types on the other axis (**_biological, psychological and social_**). This is formally introduced in Chapter 6 on Resilience and Risk (*see* Table 6.3), but we give an illustrative case example in Box 3.5.

BOX 3.5 Case Example

Deepak is eight years old and his behaviour at school is giving concern to his mother, Alisha, and staff at his school. The school's special needs coordinator asks the primary mental health worker to see Deepak.

The primary mental health worker asks his mother for examples of Deepak's 'challenging behaviours'. Deepak's mother says that he behaves well at home for his father, but less so for her; he responds well to certain teachers at school, while clashing with others.

The primary mental health worker takes a developmental and family history. Pregnancy and birth were unremarkable, and Deepak was a quiet baby in his first year. He had some delay in speech and language, which the speech and language therapist, who saw him at the age of four years, said was due to a combination of receptive and expressive language delay.

Observation in the clinic suggests he is very shy and will not separate from his mother, so an individual interview is not an option. Deepak however volunteers that things have become worse since he had a new teacher who is constantly telling him off and blaming him when things don't go right.

The primary mental health worker visits the school to observe Deepak in the classroom. This reveals that Deepak has difficulty following his class teacher's instructions, but if the classroom teaching assistant explains things to him carefully, he can concentrate well and will eventually complete the task set, although he is struggling with writing. In the playground, he is observed to be eager to play with others, who do not seem as keen to play with him. Deepak seems unable to kick a ball straight: it always seems to go in the wrong place.

Based on this initial collection of impressions from a variety of sources, the primary mental health worker fills in the four-P grid (*see* Table 3.1). She then discusses this with the school special needs coordinator, and they agree a plan. The primary mental health worker will get Deepak assessed by the paediatric occupational therapist and reassessed by the speech and language therapist; and the special needs coordinator will prioritise Deepak for assessment by the school's educational psychologist.

These assessments subsequently confirm their suspicions: Deepak is struggling in the classroom due to a combination of continuing language difficulties, below-average intellectual ability and dyspraxia. He is given extra special needs input, has more one-to-one support from the classroom assistant, and changes class to be with a teacher who is very gentle with him. Although Deepak still finds school a challenging place to be, the extra support helps him cope better and feel more positive about his achievements. His parents are very relieved that at last they and the school staff understand enough about the nature of Deepak's problems to be able to do something about them.

Involving the child in the assessment

A child should be helped to feel *involved* in what is going on from the start. Introductions and explanations of who you are and how he got to meet you should be

TABLE 3.1 Four-P grid applied to Case Example in Box 3.5

	Biological	Psychological	Social
Predisposing (Vulnerability factors)	Deepak has delayed receptive and expressive language	He tends to clash with mother	
Precipitating (Trigger factors)	He struggles with writing He cannot kick a ball	Deepak feels victimised by his new class teacher	Deepak has recently started a new school year
Perpetuating (Maintaining factors)		The more he gets behind, the more he feels it's not worth trying	Deepak is having difficulty making lasting friendships
Protective (Resilience)		Deepak can try hard to please others Deepak's mother is keen to get him help	He has an intact two-parent family with two supportive parents

directed at the child, in age-appropriate language. Explanations delivered only to parents are not sufficient. The child can then be involved in a discussion, with parents present and contributing as necessary, for as long as he is able. Younger children will often be more interested in playing with the available toys or drawing materials, but most will still listen. The child can then join in the conversation again when he wants, or when you involve him again.

Most children in this age range prefer to be seen *with at least one parent* initially, but there may be some situations when you decide to start the interview with the child alone (such as when there is alleged abuse, or when the parent has so many complaints about the child that it is painful to have the child present, so you decide to see each of them separately). It is helpful to have several techniques available for drawing the child into the conversation, whether or not the parent is present.

A useful place to start is to ask the child whether he knows *what has made people worried* about him – and who he thinks is most worried. This reveals his view and how much he is aware of his parent's concerns. An inhibited answer to this question may indicate the child's anxiety about:

➤ your response – perhaps you are going to tell him off
➤ his parent's response – perhaps she will be cross or upset
➤ the situation
➤ things in general.

An alternative cause of an inhibited answer relates to language: English may not be his first language; or he may have a language delay or disorder; or he may have a learning disability. Such difficulties may or may not be recognised: at any rate, you may not be aware of them before you begin the interview.

A child may need your help to become more **relaxed**, or reassurance that he will not be told off and that there are no right or wrong answers – you just want to know what he thinks. Getting down onto the child's level and playing or sharing a drawing may help the child warm up, whether or not the parents remain present. A good starting point can be either drawing a **family tree** together, or asking the child to draw a picture of who is in his family. You can then talk about the family, prompting if necessary with questions such as: 'Who do people say you are most like?', 'Who do you play with most?' or 'Who do you get on with best?' Asking the child the age of both parents can generate a laugh or two and act as an ice-breaker, partly because younger children often get this wildly wrong. The child's version of what jobs parents have outside home may be as interesting as the adult answer. A child can usually give some information about grandparents, such as how close they live and how often they are involved, and it is helpful to know what he calls them (nan, nanny, grandma, granny . . .). Younger children can be involved in playing with toy figures in the room if these are available, and if appropriate can be asked who the figures represent. Older children can be asked to draw a timeline showing either recent salient events or the life changes that have occurred since birth.

Such **participative tasks** can give the child a role, help him feel useful, make him more relaxed, provide an opportunity for adult approval and build up a positive relationship with the professional as well as provide valuable information about how the child sees things.

A useful **question** to ask everyone at an early stage is **what they hope to achieve from you as a professional, or the service you represent**. You may need to caution them to be realistic about this. You can then agree realistic goals for the assessment – or the package of assessment and treatment that your service could provide. Don't forget to include the child in this discussion.

Alternatively, you can ask everyone to be unrealistic, by posing the '**miracle question**', which was developed in solution-focused family therapy. You ask each family member to imagine that while he or she is asleep at night, a miracle happens that results in all their problems (or at least the ones that brought them to this assessment) magically resolving. When the family member wakes up, what does he notice has changed? You may need to pursue this in some detail to extract the maximum benefit from it. The miracle question provides a positive way of stating the family's discontents, and can lead on to an exploration of exceptions: When are things all right? For instance, what about the times when Jack does what he is told first time, instead of having a tantrum because he has been asked *not* to do something? What is different about these occasions? Is there any strategy here that can be built on?

The '**three wishes**' question is particularly useful in the individual interview, but can also be used with parents present or can be directed at parents too. 'If I had a magic wand and could grant you three wishes, what would they be?' The answer may just include material things, but this can be explored to elicit some of the child's beliefs and attitudes. Setting a time limit to this question such as: 'The wishes have to be used in the next five minutes – otherwise they will disappear' avoids the whole of your assessment time being taken up by this question. Other answers may reveal something more surprising, such as:

➤ mum to stop worrying so much
➤ to stop having bad dreams and scary thoughts
➤ to stop being bullied at school
➤ to be better at physical education
➤ mum and dad to stop arguing (the child may be afraid to say this if a parent is present).

Seeing the child alone should always be considered and is good practice, as many children are more forthcoming when seen on their own. It could be counterproductive or even unethical to insist that a child sees you alone if he expresses a clear wish not to. Sometimes this can be overcome by waiting until the child is more familiar with you or by asking a colleague (perhaps of a different gender) who has not met either parent to see the child alone. In any case, the child's wishes should be respected (as long as they really are the child's wishes and not just the parent's idea of the child's wishes).

There may be various reasons making a child reluctant to talk about things with a parent present. For instance:

➤ he may not want his parents to be aware of how he feels
➤ he may not want his parents to know something he has done
➤ he may not want his parents to know something someone else has done
➤ he may be afraid of saying something that might make a parent upset, cross or worried
➤ he may not want his parents to know that he knows something
➤ he may experience a parent as interrupting or taking over the conversation.

BOX 3.6 Practice Points for assessment

Remember that all children develop at different rates, leading to huge variations between individuals.
Try to clarify who wants what and why now?
Look at the presenting problem in the light of the child's development.
Try to understand the family and cultural context.
Gather as much information as possible about the child from a variety of sources.
Involve the child in the assessment process.
Share your initial thoughts with the family.

Interviewing preadolescent children

If you decide to see the child on his own, explain to his parent(s) that it is something you do routinely. Ask the child if it is all right for his parents to leave the room for a bit; if the child is adamantly against this idea, then it would be unwise to force things, and better to wait until he is more comfortable with this prospect.

Observe how the child separates, and how parent(s) deal with this. Tell the child what you do and don't know; children often assume that professionals know all about their problems (he may by now have heard what his parents have told you). Consider what to say about confidentiality, but mentioning that there are some things you may *have* to tell parents can be an awkward beginning to any interview.

There are several things that can be done in an individual interview with a child. The fact that you are doing it at all indicates that you are taking the child seriously. The answers to questions may provide important information that could not be obtained in any other way.

BOX 3.7 Case Example

> When seen alone as part of a routine assessment, Jim, aged seven years, mentions that he has seen his mother's boyfriend slap his elder sister round the face. There has been no previous mention of this man.

The style and content of an interview with a child depends upon not only the child's developmental stage but also **the reason for meeting with the child**. This may be one or more of the following:
➤ to discover facts that only the child knows
➤ to reveal at least part of the child's emotional state
➤ to observe language, social or cognitive functioning.

Question-and-answer interviews are quite adequate for children aged seven years and over, but it is helpful to have felt-tips, paper and imaginative toys available. In the under-sevens, observing a child's drawings or play may be used as a substitute for interview, but don't read too much into drawings or representational play without confirmation from the child. Other useful **observations** can be done without seeing the child alone: for instance focusing on the child's level of attention and hyperactivity, or the child's interaction with siblings or parents. These are more likely to be natural if the child is relaxed by being pleasurably occupied with play or drawing materials.

If you decide to do a talking interview, it is crucial to take into account how children's differences from adults are likely to affect the interview.
➤ *Children think in a wholly different manner from adults* and do not have the capacity for abstract conceptualisation that comes naturally to an adult professional; they are of necessity bound to the specific, concrete and particular. Encourage the child to tell you if he does not understand your question!
➤ *Children have little concept of therapeutic contracts and doctor-patient relationships*; they may well not understand why you are asking particular questions, nor what sort of answers they are supposed to supply. Or they may assume that you are going to prod them or give them an injection (whether you are a doctor or not)!

Support a child's attempts to communicate. Be friendly. Sit down, or get to the same level in some way. Try to talk *with* rather than talk *at*: use simple words and ideas; check the child understands your questions; exaggerate your facial expressions and tone of voice; show interest in his responses. Beware of teases or jokes that may be misunderstood. Allow the child time to respond.

An interview to discover facts that only the child knows

➤ Explain what you are going to ask about:
'I want to know something about the pain in your tummy.'
'Let's talk about what made you cross last time you had a temper.'
➤ Start with neutral conversation topics such as his hobbies or interests to establish a conversation. Move on to more loaded topics later. If you sense the child's anxiety or embarrassment is inhibiting him, move back to a more neutral topic.
➤ Ask very specific questions that do not require any generalisations: 'The very last time you took something that wasn't yours . . . tell me when it was and what happened . . .' is preferable to asking, 'How often do you steal?', and 'What is the name of your best friend?' is better than asking, 'Do you have lots of friends?'

An interview to ascertain emotional state

➤ Explain that you want to know something about the child's thoughts and feelings and are going to ask questions about them.
➤ Start with a relatively neutral area. If this is school, ask: 'Which school do you go to? What year are you in? What's the name of your teacher?' in order to set the scene.
➤ Then say:
'Most children have things they like about school and things they don't like. What do you like about your school? What's your favourite subject? What are you best at? What things don't you like? Is there anyone you don't like?' The idea is to provide the child with practice talking about their own responses and feelings.
➤ Give legitimacy to feelings by prefacing some questions with remarks like: 'Many children have . . .' or 'A girl I once knew . . .' For instance, it might be appropriate to proceed with:
'A lot of children feel very cross with their brothers when they do some things and feel very nice towards them when they do other things. What sort of things does your brother do? How do you feel about that?'
➤ Because most preadolescent children have rather poor vocabularies with which to describe feelings and relationships, it may be appropriate to put questions in a multiple-choice format, in order to indicate to the child the range of responses expected and the words that might be used:
'When your father left home and went away, I wonder how you felt?' [Pause to see if a reply is forthcoming.]
'You might have felt pleased, or you might have felt sad. Some boys would have felt frightened or cross or had some different sort of feeling. Others have lots of different feelings. How about you?'
Use of '. . . some different sort of feeling' allows for the possibility of an unexpected emotional response. If some open-choice statement such as this is not included, the child may feel there are some thoughts and feelings he is not allowed to express.

Interviews as an opportunity to observe language, social or cognitive functioning

➤ During the interview, clinical observations about the form rather than the content of the child's responses can provide information about language development, capacity to relate to adults, level of intelligence and, if a drawing or a piece of writing is requested, fine motor coordination.

BOX 3.8 Case Example

A seven-year-old girl, Lucy, is brought to you by her mother. The school complains that she is very withdrawn in class, but her mother claims there is very little wrong at home. Mother does not want a referral to specialist CAMHS. You ask the mother to leave you alone for ten minutes, and explain to Lucy that her mother says people at school are worried about her, and you want to know what she thinks. Initially, she seems very shy, so you provide her some felt tips and paper, and you both sit on the floor. You ask her to draw who is at home, and she immediately tells you how much she misses her father, who left three months ago ...

Making the assessment therapeutic

Sharing your understanding of the presenting problem with the parent(s) – and if possible, the children – can lead to a joint *formulation*. This is simply a summary of the information obtained that can take the form of a descriptive summary or a four-P grid or both. Family members may find relief in having an explanation of the child's difficulties. They may be able to target perpetuating factors if the predisposing and precipitating factors are too difficult to alter, or build on the protective factors or solutions identified during your assessment. In some cases, no further management is necessary: understanding what makes the child behave in this way at this time is helpful enough in itself.

BOX 3.9 Summary of important components of an assessment

The presenting problem
- *Who* sees *what* as a problem?
- Why *this* problem in *this* child at *this* time?
- Examples of the problem
- Is it within the normal range of development?

The developmental history
- Birth
- First year
- Milestones
- Toddlerhood
- Nursery
- School
- Medical history

The family history (maximise the input from the child)
- Siblings
- Parents
- Grandparents
- Absent members of the nuclear family
- Other important carers

Optional extras in the history
- Daily eating pattern
- Weekly exercise pattern
- Impact of the presenting problem (on each family member)
- Protective factors
- Beliefs or attitudes relevant to the presenting problem
- What exceptions are there to the problem?
- What solutions have been found so far?
- What was happening for each parent when the same age as the child is now?

Ways of involving the child
- See the child with a familiar adult initially
- Start by directing introductory comments at the child
- Balance verbal and non-verbal interactions with the child, according to developmental age
- Choose participative tasks such as drawing the family or playing with toy figures
- Pace your questions according to the child's developmental stage and readiness to engage
- Choose questions that involve the child such as the miracle question or three wishes
- Talk (or play) exclusively with the child even though other family members are present
- See the child on his own

Observation
- Child's level of activity and concentration
- Child's ability to communicate verbally and non-verbally
- Child's relationship with carer
- (Each) carer's attitude to child
- Child's relationship with you – initially and after warm-up

Other sources of information
- Talking to various combinations of family members
- Talking to other adults involved with the child
- Obtaining information (as a letter, by telephone or by e-mail) from other professionals who know the child and family
- Observation in different contexts of the child and/or other family members

Summarising
- Fill in a four-P grid
- Generate a formulation
- Share your thoughts with family members to help decide on an action plan

BOX 3.10 Alarm Bells that may emerge during assessment which may need further exploration

---

Parental issues
- Parental mental health difficulties
- Parental substance misuse
- Domestic violence
- Harsh interaction with the child in the room

Child issues
- Separation anxiety
- Lack of social activities
- Poor sleep
- Failure to engage with the professional in conversation, drawing or play

School issues
- Bullying
- Not coping with schoolwork

MANAGEMENT AND PREVENTION

Parents have a key role in promoting healthy development and the emotional well-being of children and young people – but so do a range of agencies and professionals working with children, especially schools. There are plentiful government guidance documents and initiatives of relevance, including NICE guidelines,[13,14] Social and Emotional Aspects of Learning[15], Healthy Schools[16] and Targeted Mental Health in Schools.[17] The various ways in which child mental health professionals can play a part in this are summarised in Box 3.11, and then described in more detail in the following sections.

BOX 3.11 Ways of promoting children's development and emotional well-being

---

Provide age-appropriate information and advice
- Share your understanding (formulation)
- Discuss child development
- Provide written information and advice
- Recommend where to find further information (such as the resources listed below)
- Give a book prescription if available

Consider ongoing support and advice for the child and/or family
- About specific problems (*see* individual chapters in this book)
- About developmental changes
- From local services
- From national or local charities and parent support groups
- From government advice websites

Promoting healthy lifestyles
- Advice about diet and exercise (*see* Chapter 44)
- Sex education – follow the child's lead by answering his questions openly in language he can understand
- Encourage regular dental check-ups
- Encourage checks of vision and hearing, particularly if there are any concerns and these have not been done recently
- Reinforce any medical advice given by a general practitioner or paediatrician

Promoting cognitive development
- Encourage (parents to encourage) the child to learn through imaginative play and exploring the world around him
- Encourage (parents to encourage) the child to pursue a range of activities and interests

Promoting psychosocial development
- Encourage parents to give the child age-appropriate responsibilities
- Encourage parents to explore opportunities for the child to meet children of the same age and make friends
- Encourage (the child to join) after-school clubs and other group activities
- Encourage parents and other involved adults to provide good role-models for the child
- Discuss online safety and Internet friendships

Information and advice

Information and explanation may be enough to help parents understand the child better, and thereby cope more effectively – for instance by appreciating expected developmental changes or empathising with the child's point of view. The professional can helpfully combine this with suggestions about how to encourage the child's positive development.

BOX 3.12 Case Example

When Lucy is seven years old, her mother asks to see the community school nurse to discuss Lucy's anxiety about going to birthday parties with her school friends. The community school nurse asks about Lucy's social experiences, and discovers that she is an only child whose main playmates so far have been a next-door neighbour and a cousin, both of roughly the same age. With mother's permission, she checks with Lucy's class teacher, who says that Lucy is fairly confident in class, answering questions when asked, and is well able to do joint tasks when paired with another pupil but seems a bit shy when in group situations, and does not usually volunteer her views in group discussions. Academically, Lucy is achieving in the average range for everything.

The community school nurse arranges to see both Lucy's parents. She tells them that as far as she can tell, Lucy is making satisfactory developmental progress. She could benefit from some more opportunity to develop her social skills, particularly in situations involving more than one other child. They discuss possible ways to achieve this, and brainstorm various possibilities, including after-school clubs, Brownies, swimming lessons, dancing classes and horse-riding lessons. They then involve Lucy in the discussion, and ask her to choose one or two group activities to try first. She says she would like to learn to ride a horse, and would also like to join the church choir (which her parents haven't thought of).

Lucy's parents do not make her go to birthday parties until she feels ready. She makes new friends through the choir and the horse-riding and invites them home, as well as some of her friends from school. Six months later, she announces that she would really like to go to the birthday party of a friend at school who does the same horse-riding class; by then, she knows several of the children invited to the party.

Reassurance and advice may be supplemented by *information from other sources*, such as locally produced leaflets, books for loan (in some areas called 'biblio-therapy' or book prescription schemes) or the Internet. The plethora of available information may be confusing, and some websites may contradict others, so some guidance may be needed on what is most likely to be helpful. A few suggestions are given in the Resources section at the end of this chapter.

Support
Asking for help may not be easy. A parent may feel:
➤ ashamed
➤ embarrassed
➤ that if things have got bad enough to ask for help, then it must be all her fault
➤ that she has failed as a parent in some way.

Recognising when help is needed and having the courage to admit this is the most responsible thing a parent can do. Seeking advice and support at an early stage can prevent a problem become entrenched or escalating. So parents should be praised for having the wisdom and courage to seek help.

It may be helpful to use the analogy of a physical symptom such as pain that may be a sign of trouble developing and should be diagnosed and treated early to prevent becoming worse and causing long-term difficulties. Many child mental health conditions are *easier to treat earlier rather than later* in the course of their development: examples include phobias, school refusal, chronic fatigue syndrome, obsessive-compulsive disorder, ADHD and behaviour problems. It is part of the purpose of this book to enable front-line practitioners (Tier 1 or universal services) to catch such conditions at an early stage so that interventions can be provided without having to wait for specialised services (Tier 3 or targeted services) to become involved (*see* Chapter 1 on Context).

It may become evident from your assessment that the main caregiver is relatively isolated and could do with some *support*, either practical or emotional or

both. This may be available from various sources, but you may need to help facilitate this by involving:
➤ another caregiver or the other parent
➤ a grandparent or member of extended family
➤ a family friend
➤ a children or family centre
➤ a parent support group
➤ a behaviour management training group
➤ a family support worker.

Information on what is available locally can often be obtained from the health visitor, community school nurse, social services, the local library, the local Citizens Advice Bureau, the child's school, a local health centre or national websites (*see* the end of this chapter).

BOX 3.13 Case Example

Jasvinder is an isolated mother with an eight-year-old son, Dilip, who has been assessed as having dyspraxia and specific literacy difficulties. His behaviour can be quite challenging and would be exhausting for most mothers to cope with, but he has begun to manage better at school now that he is receiving special needs input. He is an only child. His father can manage him much more easily, but he works long hours, so is available to play with Dilip and take him out only on Sundays.

The community school nurse has been aware of Dilip's behaviour problems for some time through her conversations with the school special needs coordinator, but it is not until Jasvinder asks Dilip's class teacher for help that the community school nurse gets involved. She arranges to meet Jasvinder at home during the day, while Dilip is at school. It emerges that Jasvinder has had no contact with her parents since marrying a man they did not approve of. Her only sister agreed to an arranged marriage, and lives close to their parents, so – in contrast – enjoys their support. The community school nurse explores what has made Jasvinder ask for help now, rather than earlier. Jasvinder explains that she used to see a lot of her only brother, but he has recently returned to India.

The community school nurse brainstorms with Jasvinder a variety of supports that she might feel able to access. Eventually, they agree that Jasvinder will attend an Asian women's group, but only if the Community School Nurse arranges a meeting to introduce Jasvinder to the two Asian family support workers who run this group.

Jasvinder starts attending this group. Through the people she meets there, she starts some voluntary work for a local Asian charity set up to support the victims of family ostracism (including those who have escaped threatened honour killings). She subsequently takes up paid part-time employment with this organisation, which results in her establishing a wide social circle of other Asian women, and also offering support to Asian women who have had similar experiences.

Jasvinder still finds Dilip's behaviour challenging, but this no longer concerns her as much, and she gradually finds it easier to be calm and firm with him.

Physical health

Good physical health is important for good mental health at any age. Children are often brought to a mental health professional with emotional or behavioural symptoms that are a consequence of **an illness or chronic disorder**. It is important to check that this is receiving adequate attention. A common example used to be constipation and the resultant faecal incontinence, which used often to be referred initially to CAMHS: now it should be clear that paediatric assessment and treatment should be tried first (*see* Chapter 24 on Faecal Incontinence). Another example is any developmental disability, such as cerebral palsy, dyspraxia or developmental delay of unknown origin.

As this is the age range when children lose their milk teeth and acquire their secondary dentition, regular attendance at a **dentist** is important. This will not only help maintain the function of the teeth they have, but should also develop the habit of going to the dentist as a positive experience. Children who attend the dentist only when there is a painful procedure to be done are at risk of developing a dental phobia.

As **puberty** begins during or at the end of middle childhood, it is important for children to have some knowledge about this before it occurs – otherwise the physical changes that occur can be experienced as confusing or in some cases frightening. Most socially aware children will get some sort of knowledge from their peers, but this may vary in its accuracy and completeness.

BOX 3.14 Case Example

> Father to 11-year-old son: 'Now it's time for us to do some sex education.'
> Son: 'OK, dad, what do you want to know?'

There is debate about when and whether **sex education** should be carried out, and if so whether by schools or parents. The authors' view is that children's questions about sex should be answered as soon as they are able to understand the answers, which in practice means as soon as they start asking questions about it. These are most likely to come up in conversation with parents who make themselves approachable, or in the context of Personal, Social and Health Education lessons in school. Ideally, discussions should be held before any classmates start entering puberty, which means by the age of eight years and before or during school year four. Sex education should preferably come from both sources (home and school) and continue for the remaining two years of primary school. Leaving it to secondary school risks leaving it too late – until after children's views have been formed by other sources of information, such as peer discussions, teen magazines, or websites. It is not just a matter of imparting dry facts: the 'facts' are best learnt in the context of a discussion in which children feel able to ask questions, and the discussion can be combined with a debate about the nature of relationships and the variety of relevant cultural or religious attitudes and moral beliefs.

Cognitive development

Concerns about a child's learning or progress at school should be discussed initially with his teachers. However, parents may seek advice from others if they are worried that their child seems immature for her age or different from her peers or is struggling to learn to read or write. A child who is struggling to keep up with her peers due to a specific or generalised learning difficulty may be compliant but withdrawn ('no trouble') in class – particularly girls – or have a behaviour problem and disruptive influence for no apparent reason – particularly boys (see the distinction between externalising and internalising above, in the introductory section on psychosocial development). Alternatively, there may be a mismatch between the child's (average range) ability and parental expectations.

BOX 3.15 Case Example

Matilda, aged seven years, seems unhappy when she gets home from school. Her parents ask her if she is being bullied, but she says not. When they talk to Matilda's class teacher, she says Matilda is no trouble in class, behaves very well, always does as she is told, and seems to get on with her work. Matilda's parents ask to see what work she has done and find a sheaf of drawings, but not much else. The teacher says that she has observed Matilda playing happily in the playground during break time, and she seems to have several friends, though none of them particularly close.

In the National Curriculum Standard Assessment Tests (SATs),[18] Matilda scores below average in all subjects. Her parents involve the Parent Partnership service and ask for her to be tested. The school special needs coordinator is able to arrange for a trainee educational psychologist currently attached to the school to do the Wechsler Intelligence Scale for Children (version IV). This shows that Matilda's overall functioning is just above the moderate learning difficulties range (full scale intelligence quotient in the range 68–76); she has a relatively even profile, without any outstanding strengths or weaknesses.

Her parents then involve Parent Partnership again in meeting with the class teacher and special needs coordinator. This meeting leads to an agreement that Matilda will be placed on 'School Action Plus' and get a differentiated work set and input from a learning support assistant, whom she will share with other pupils.

A term later, Matilda's parents realise that she has been much happier on her return from school. She has even been able to ask a friend home from school occasionally.

Reading difficulties can be prevented in most children by a combination of:
➤ reading stories to the child from an early age
➤ making reading materials seem interesting, including not only picture books for younger children but also, when the child is ready, comics, factual books relating to the child's particular interests or strategy books (with clues leading from one page to another)

➤ involving the child in reading as part of everyday activities, such as reading advertisements, playing word games or word searches together or reading maps
➤ using educational computer games that involve reading as part of the fun activity.

Some children may struggle with some or all of these activities, and in extreme cases (such as in Box 3.16) may develop an aversion to any reading tasks, which can make it very difficult for a parent to back up the school's efforts by encouraging reading practice at home. Such children may require specialised input from a learning support assistant and/or special needs teacher at school.

Parents can similarly encourage spelling, writing and numeracy by integrating them into fun activities at home, in addition to helping the child complete homework. Some parents may find this easier than others, perhaps through differences in motivation, cultural attitudes to education or ability: a parent may have her own learning difficulties that make it difficult for her to encourage her child in educational activities. Parents should if possible work closely with the class teacher or the school's special needs coordinator to identify any specific difficulties at an early stage and obtain appropriate special needs help. There may be a role for the child mental health professional in encouraging parents to work closely with teachers, or alternatively the Parent Partnership Team or Parent Support and Advisory Service may be able to fulfil this role. It is important for the child to hear the same messages from school and parents, and a collaborative relationship between home and school is likely to be far more constructive for the child than an adversarial relationship.

BOX 3.16 Case Examples

> Tyrone, an eight-year-old black Afro-Caribbean boy, is a well-known troublemaker in his school. His class teacher suggests his mother, Jemima, should get some help, so she sees her general practitioner, who asks the primary mental health worker to see him.
>
> When they meet, Jemima explains that she does not have many problems with Tyrone at home, except when she asks him to read! Tyrone's class teacher keeps phoning her about his disruptive behaviour in lessons and she feels as if she is expecting her to do something about it. She feels that the school blames her for his poor reading; the teachers ask her to help him with his reading homework, but he hates it and screams if she tries to encourage him to read any book. In contrast, he enjoys his mathematics and art homework. He also enjoys playing football in a club at weekends and helping his father with carpentry at home. He gets on well enough with his 12-year-old sister, who is doing well at her secondary school.
>
> As Tyrone's problems appear to be mainly based at school, the primary mental health worker, with mother's permission, asks his teachers how he is getting on at school. They are concerned about Tyrone's disruptive behaviour in lessons and think it is impairing his learning; they are critical of his parents for not getting him to do any reading at home. He did well in his mathematics Standard Assessment Tests (SATs)

but his scores for reading and spelling were very low, and he is not getting much written work done in class or at home. He very much enjoys art lessons and maths and concentrates well in these.

The primary mental health worker explains to the school's special needs coordinator that Tyrone's mother is really struggling to get him to read at home but finds his behaviour at other times relatively easy to manage. They arrange for him to have an assessment of his literacy skills by a specialist teacher, who identifies that Tyrone has a specific literacy difficulty, and then suggests that this may be causing Tyrone's difficult behaviour in class, rather than the other way round.

Tyrone's Individual Education Plan (IEP) is amended and he is placed on the school's special needs register at the level of 'School Action Plus'. He is given extra support in the form of small-group withdrawal teaching in literacy skills and a share in a classroom learning support assistant in lessons that require him to read or write. Over the next school year, his behaviour continues to be challenging at times, but his parents are very relieved to have an explanation for Tyrone's behavioural difficulties, and now work closely with the school to manage these. They pay for one lesson per week from a specialised dyslexia teacher, which they manage to fit around his football club on Saturdays. This teacher is able to give Tyrone's parents ways of gently encouraging his reading at home, including the use of comics and children's graphic novels. Tyrone's mother teaches him to touch-type, so he can produce written homework tidily – but she is not able to persuade the school to allow Tyrone to use a laptop in school until the following school year. Tyrone's parents also work hard to build up his self-esteem by giving him lots of opportunities to improve in football and carpentry, and by enrolling him in a karate class, where he seems to be able to express some of his frustrations in a controlled way.

Psychosocial development

Being able to get on with and relate to others involves a number of skills including:
➤ an ability to see things from another person's perspective
➤ the ability to make new friendships and sustain them
➤ the ability to approach a new problem in a way that is likely to lead to a solution
➤ the ability to approach conflict in a way that is likely to lead to a resolution.

These skills can be taught by teachers in Personal and Social Education lessons, where role-plays or discussion of hypothetical problem scenarios may help. Parents may be able to help by monitoring the child's interactions with others, and prompting when necessary to develop pro-social skills. Most children learn many of these skills without being formally taught them, through their interactions with other children, either on the playground, with siblings or cousins, or in their neighbourhood. Children with Autistic Spectrum Disorders (*see* Chapter 32) may find all these skills difficult to acquire; many other children may benefit from help to improve some or all of these abilities (*see* Case Example in Box 3.17).

BOX 3.17 Case Example

Daniel, aged nine years, is in Year 5 at his primary school, and is in trouble for fighting. The social inclusion pupil support worker agrees to see him at the request of the class teacher, who explains that she is not worried about his behaviour in the classroom, which is generally calm and compliant. He is an average pupil, can concentrate well, and is keeping up with reading, spelling, writing and mathematics. He is able to work well with one other pupil, who is his best friend, but he seems to clash very easily with others, particularly in unstructured situations such as the playground, the lunch queue or on the way to and from school. The social inclusion support worker obtains parental consent to see him on his own.

She discusses the last time he had a fight with someone. Daniel explains that Vikesh tried to take his football away from him. She enquires further. Daniel says he was in the playground with a school football, trying to start up his own football game, wishing he could be part of the football game that some others had just started with another ball. She asks him what he thought Vikesh was doing. He said he thought Vikesh was trying to take the ball away from him so that he couldn't play with it. She asks Daniel what he thinks goes on in football.

He says, 'People kick the ball into the goal'.

'How do they get near the goal?'

'By dribbling it there', Daniel says.

She prompts him.

'And by passing it to someone else.'

'So what happens if someone wants to stop you getting the ball near the goal?'

'They run so fast they take over the ball before it gets to the other person.'

'Or ... ?'

'Or someone tackles.'

'So do you think Vikesh might have been trying to start a game with you by tackling you?'

Daniel admits he hadn't thought of that.

When they discuss other examples of fights that Daniel has got into, it emerges that he often misinterprets the actions of others in this way, and that once he has got into a situation he is unhappy with, he doesn't know how to get out of it except to feel cross with the other pupil (because it must be the other's fault) and start a fight with him in order to punish him (it is usually a boy).

Over the next three sessions of seeing Daniel on his own, the social inclusion support worker explores Daniel's interpretations of others' social approaches, and helps him see there may be several possible explanations for the way another child whom he doesn't know well behaves towards him. Daniel explores social situations by drawing pictures of them, with thought bubbles for what people might be thinking. She also introduces some problem-solving techniques, and brainstorms ways that Daniel can make things all right with others when they seem to have gone wrong.

Gradually, Daniel's fighting becomes less frequent, and he is able to make more friends, although many of the other pupils are still a bit wary of him and tend to avoid him. After five sessions, the social inclusion support worker reports back to the class teacher and Daniel's mother that she thinks he has been able to absorb what they have discussed. She agrees to have only one more meeting for the time being, to explain to Daniel that she thinks he has done so well that he can manage things on his own from now on.

Other ways in which parents or other involved adults (or older siblings) can *encourage psychosocial development* include the following.

➤ *Maintain a secure base*. A child is unlikely to make successful forays into new social contexts unless he feels comfortable with his relationships at home. A safe foundation for exploring new relationships can be provided by at least one core relationship with someone who can:
  — be there when needed
  — comfort when hurt
  — be available to listen
  — provide a safe place to talk about experiences, thoughts or feelings
  — be as calm and non-judgmental as possible
  — praise and encourage as much as possible
  — provide advice or practical support when needed.
➤ *Model pro-social behaviours* in the family or in other contexts where adults are in a position of authority:
  — demonstrate positive (affirming, praising) rather than negative (critical, moaning) attitudes and interactions
  — provide a model of how to express emotions
  — provide a model of how to cope with success or adversity
  — express values and morals, providing guidance when necessary.
➤ Give gradually increasing *responsibilities* in the home environment:
  — chores in the home, such as laying the table, washing up or sweeping mess off the floor
  — looking after a pet
  — helping to look after a younger sibling.
➤ Provide *positive feedback* for even small successes to build up confidence and a sense of achievement.
➤ Search out *opportunities for social interaction* with peers and positive adult role models, in addition to school:
  — informal activities with friends, such as kicking a ball around in the park or playing chasing games
  — slightly more organised activities requiring some adult supervision, such as going swimming with friends or visiting an animal sanctuary
  — organised team games such as football, hockey or cricket – some children may feel less anxious in team sports than individual
  — organised individual or group sport lessons, such as tennis, swimming, athletics or martial arts – other children may prefer activities involving solitary activity, highly structured interaction or parallel play rather than repeated unpredictable interactions in a group context

   — organised clubs providing a variety of activities, such as cubs, scouts, brownies, or other youth clubs.

➤ Some children who are shy or socially anxious may require more ***encouragement*** than others. This may involve being accompanied by a familiar adult, at least initially, to activities that are novel or frightening. It is important to arrange things so that the child is able to experience social successes, and then build on these. Parents may encounter some resistance, and may need to find a way of persisting with an introduction to a new social situation without forcing the child into something arousing vehement opposition.

➤ Adult ***supervision*** may be necessary, particularly for younger children, when embarking on new social ventures.

➤ ***Schools*** can promote psychosocial development in a number of ways, in addition to the daily interactions that are an essential part of school life. Coordination between parents and school staff may be important for children who are struggling with social interactions, and can enable parents to receive feedback on the child's progress. Examples include:

   — lunchtime clubs
   — after-school clubs
   — circle time
   — peer mentoring by an older pupil
   — a buddy system using children in the same year
   — a robust anti-bullying policy
   — a culture in which teachers listen to pupils and pupils expect that teachers will listen to them.

BOX 3.18 Practice Points for management

Normalise the child's presenting problem if it is within the range of normal development.
Ensure that parents have access to any necessary ***information***.
Help the parent(s) engage with any available sources of ***support***, for instance within the extended family or other parents
Ensure that any ***paediatric*** issues are attended to.
Are ***checks*** of hearing, vision and teeth up to date?
Can ***sleep*** be improved by attention to sleep hygiene? (*See* Chapter 36 on Sleep Problems.)
Are there opportunities for improvements in ***diet***?
Are there opportunities for increasing regular ***exercise***? (*See* Chapter 44 on Diet and Exercise.)
Can a parent support the work of the class teacher more effectively by helping the child more with ***homework*** – or with non-homework educational activities? Is the parent able to do this?
Can the working relationship between ***parents and teachers*** be improved?
Are there opportunities for the child to ***meet more children*** of a similar age?
Can the child develop ***socially and emotionally*** in other ways?

REFERRAL

Depending on the outcome of your assessment and the management options available to you, referral for further assessment or management may be in the child's best interests. Examples of others who may be able to take things further include not only specialist CAMHS but also community paediatrics, educational psychology, paediatric dietetics, paediatric occupational therapy and speech and language therapy.

Most children are screened for developmental problems in the preschool years, and screening for developmental problems should continue into the school years. However, it is important not to forget that ***sensory problems*** may not be obvious: for instance, glue ear is very common, and can cause inattention, deterioration in school performance or behaviour problems. If a parent has any suspicion that hearing might be impaired, refer to the local audiology clinic, where the child will receive an age-appropriate hearing test. Undetected poor vision can cause underperformance in class or headaches, so regular visual testing by an optician is also important.

RESOURCES

Books for children about emotions

- Aliki. *Feelings*. London: Greenwillow Books (HarperCollins); 2000.
  This may help children of four to eight years old articulate emotions.
- Cain BS, Patterson A. *Double-dip Feelings: stories to help children understand emotions*. 2nd ed. Washington DC: Magination Press (American Psychological Association); 2001.
  Explores the sometimes confusing way that humans can have two feelings at the same time.
- Lite L, Botelho H. *The Affirmation Web: a believe in yourself adventure*. London: Partners Publishing Group; 1997.
  Affirmations or positive statements build self-esteem and empower children to be the best they can. Readers follow a girl and her animal friends as they weave the Affirmation Web. They learn to believe in themselves while replacing negative messages with positive self-talk.
- Marcus IW, Marcus P, Jeschke S. *Into the Great Forest: a story for children away from parents for the first time*. Washington DC: Magination Press (American Psychological Association); 1992.
  This story for children of four to eight years is a dream adventure in which a young boy overcomes his fears about his first day at school.
- Oram H, Kitamura S. *Angry Arthur*. London: Andersen Press; 2008.
  Arthur's mother won't let him stay up to watch television, so Arthur gets very, very angry until his anger blows the universe into little pieces.

Books for children about feeling different

- Cave K, Riddell C. *Something Else*. London: Picture Puffin; 1995.
  A little creature is ostracized despite his attempts to fit in, but his experiences enable him to be accepting of others' differences: suitable for children of four to eight years.
- Pfister M. *The Rainbow Fish*. New York: North-South Books; 2007.
  A book about a beautiful fish who learns to make friends by sharing what he prizes most, his beautiful scales: for children of four to eight years.

Books for children about sex

- Harris R, Emberley M. *Let's talk about sex.* London: Walker Books; 2010.
  A humorous, well-illustrated book about growing up, changing bodies, sex and sexual health.
- Mayle P. *Where Did I Come From?* London: Macmillan Children's Books; 2006.
  This book will help parents share information with their children about sex and where babies come from.

Books for parents on emotions

- Eastman M. *Taming the Dragon in Your Child: solutions for breaking the cycle of family anger.* Chichester: John Wiley; 1994.
  Advice on helping children between the ages of one to 16 years manage angry feelings.
- Faber A, Mazlish E. *How to Talk So Kids Will Listen and Listen So Kids Will Talk.* London: Piccadilly Press Ltd; 2001.
  How to make relationships with children less stressful and more rewarding.
- Graham P, Hughes C. *So Young, So Sad, So Listen.* London: Gaskell; 2005.
  For parents of boys aged 5–16 years to facilitate information sharing, ways to manage sad feelings and raising self-esteem.
- Hunt C. *The Parenting Puzzle. how to get the best out of family life.* UK: Family Links; 2003.
  Advice on parenting, raising children's self-esteem, emotional literacy and developing relationships within the family.

Books for parents on confidence

- Hartley-Brewer E. *Self Esteem For Girls: 100 tips for raising happy and confident children.* London: Vermilion; 2000.
- Hartley-Brewer E. *Self Esteem For Boys: 100 Tips for raising happy and confident children.* London: Vermilion; 2000.
- Lindenfield G. *Confident Children: help children feel good about themselves.* London: Thorsons; 2000.
  This book helps parents of children of any age focus on developing the child's resilience.
- Parker J, Stimpson J, Rowe D. *Raising Happy Children: what every child needs their parents to know – from 0 to 11 years.* London: Mobius; 2004.
  This book helps parents think about a variety of issues without getting bogged down in diagnostic labels.

Books for professionals

- Cowie H, Boardman C, Barnsley J, *et al. Emotional Health and Well-Being: a practical guide for schools.* London: Sage; 2004.
- Lindon J. *Understanding Child Development: linking theory and practice.* London: Hodder Education; 2005.
- Schaffer HR. *Introducing Child Psychology.* Chichester: John Wiley and Sons; 2003.

Websites

- **Netmums:** www.netmums.com – A unique local network for parents with a wealth of information and advice on being a mum or dad in your locality.
- **Mumsnet:** A forum for information sharing and discussion between parents, with the aim to make parents' lives easier by pooling knowledge, experience and support. www.mumsnet.com

- **Family Lives** is a charity which offers support to anyone involved in caring for children. It provides a 24-hour helpline offering listening, support, information and guidance on all issues of concern. It also provides parent classes and workshops for parents to share ideas and learn new skills and a website containing a range of information, including leaflets on family related issues and an email support service. http://familylives.org.uk
- The **UK Council for Child Internet Safety (UKCCIS)** has set up a site in response to the Byron Report to help children keep safe while using the Internet. http://clickcleverclicksafe.direct.gov.uk/index.html
- **BBC Parenting**: www.bbc.co.uk/parenting

REFERENCES

1 Rogoff B, Sellers M, Pirrotta S, *et al.* Age of assignment of roles and responsibilities in children: a cross-cultural survey. *Human Development.* 1975; **18:** 353–69.
2 Piaget J. Piaget's theory. In: Mussen PH, editor. *Carmichael's Manual of Child Psychology (Volume 1).* New York, NY: Wiley; 1970. pp. 703–32.
3 Erikson EH. Eight ages of Man. *International Journal of Psychoanalysis.* 1966; **2:** 281–300.
4 Byron T. *Safer Children in a Digital World: report of the Byron Review.* London: Department for Children, Schools and Families and Department for Culture, Media and Sport; 2008. Available at: www.dcsf.gov.uk/byronreview (accessed 22 March 2011).
5 Layard R, Dunn J. *A Good Childhood: searching for values in a competitive age.* London: The Children's Society and Penguin Books; 2009. p. 55.
6 Byron T, 2008, op. cit.
7 Byron T. *Do we have safer children in a digital world? A review of progress since the 2008 Byron Review.* Department for Children, Schools and Families; 2010. Available at: www.dcsf.gov.uk/byronreview (accessed 22 March 2011).
8 www.dcsf.gov.uk/ukccis
9 Byron T, 2008, op. cit, p. 19 (Children's Call for Evidence).
10 Layard, op. cit. pp. 60–2.
11 Papadopoulos L. *Sexualisation of Young People.* London: Home Office; 2010.
12 Ibid.
13 National Institute for Health and Clinical Excellence. *Promoting children's social and emotional wellbeing in primary education.* NICE public health guidance 12. NICE: London; 2008. Available at: www.nice.org.uk/nicemedia/pdf/PH012Guidance.pdf (accessed 22 March 2011).
14 National Institute for Health and Clinical Excellence. *Promoting children's social and emotional wellbeing in secondary education.* NICE public health guidance 20. NICE: London; 2008. Available at: http://guidance.nice.org.uk/PH20/Guidance/pdf (accessed 22 March 2011).
15 Department for Children, Schools and Families. *Social and Emotional Aspects of Learning (SEAL): improving behaviour, improving learning.* London: Department for Children, Schools and Families; 2005. Available at: http://nationalstrategies.standards.dcsf.gov.uk/primary/publications/banda/seal (accessed 22 March 2011).
16 http://home.healthyschools.gov.uk
17 www.education.gov.uk/publications/standard/publicationDetail/Page1/DCSF-00784-2008
18 www.satsguide.co.uk/what_are_sats.htm

CHAPTER 4

Adolescence

INTRODUCTION

This chapter discusses this stage from a developmental perspective, focusing also on how to engage with adolescents and their families.

The word 'adolescence' may trigger anxiety, even for the most experienced worker – just as Pavlov's dogs salivated at the sound of a bell. Our culture, the media and to some extent the psychological literature have led us to believe that adolescence is a period of 'storm and stress'. Images readily spring to mind of sullen, stroppy, monosyllabic youngsters who may at times be aggressive, and therefore scary as well as deskilling. In reality, adolescents vary hugely in terms of their beliefs and attitudes, and consequently their behaviour in a clinical interview. The fearsome stereotypes probably apply only to a minority.

The potential for adolescent unhappiness should not however, be dismissed. A recent international study by UNICEF showed the UK serving its child and adolescent population least well out of 21 developed nations, worse even than the United States.[1] Those countries scoring highest for child well-being on an amalgam of 40 indicators included the Scandinavian countries, Holland, Spain and Switzerland. This has been blamed on increasing inequality.[2] The potential implications for the UK have been examined in a report by the Children's Society,[3] with suggestions about what could be done.

Nevertheless, adolescence can be one of the most varied and interesting developmental stages. It is a time of rapid change and growth which can be confusing not just for the individual but also for those around her. Presenting problems must be seen within the context of a range of factors – in addition to the adolescent's developmental stage:

➤ the individual's temperament and developing personality
➤ the individual's intellectual capacity and academic attainment
➤ the individual's emotional intelligence and social maturity
➤ family background, beliefs and culture
➤ family functioning – the inter-relationships between family members
➤ the wider environment including school, peers and group pressures
➤ the extent to which the adolescent follows her family's culture and beliefs or follows those of her peers
➤ the possible relevance of substance misuse
➤ life events.

Working with adolescents provides a great deal of variety and can be immensely rewarding, as change can often be dramatic. Working with the adolescent's family and other involved professionals can lead to even more challenges and satisfactions.

Perhaps more than at any other developmental stage, working with adolescents may bring back memories and issues from the worker's own background. For both the client and the professional, adolescence is (or has been) an opportunity to reflect upon one's emerging identity, explore relationships, question beliefs, determine values and explore one's strengths and weaknesses – all of which shape the developing personality. It is not surprising therefore that issues presented by an adolescent may resonate with issues for the professional. This process can be enriching as well as challenging.

This can also be the time when the young person feels at her most vulnerable. As an individual is developing into adulthood she is often treated by society as an adult. Possible reasons for this include: being a young carer, looking more mature than she is, or hanging out with older friends. In addition, the young person may have to cope with conflicting messages from society/parents/siblings/peers about the age at which sex, smoking, alcohol and other drugs may or may not be allowed. If a trusting relationship is developed with a professional, an adolescent may feel able to share her private anxieties, which is likely to be a tremendous relief. Examples of possible concerns follow.

➤ When am I going to start my periods?
➤ When is my pubic hair going to grow?
➤ Am I too fat or too thin?
➤ Do I want to build up my muscles and be strong, or stay puny and sensitive?
➤ Am I gay or straight?
➤ Is it evil or harmful to masturbate?
➤ How much worse are my spots going to get?
➤ My breasts are too big.
➤ My penis is too small.
➤ How could any boy possibly fancy me?
➤ How could any girl ever want to go out with me?
➤ I am never going to understand equations.
➤ I am sure all my friends think I'm stupid.
➤ Do my friends think I'm cool?
➤ Did I say the wrong thing today to that girl I fancy?
➤ Will that boy I fancy ever look at me?
➤ Does a joint make me feel better or worse?
➤ Do I enjoy the right music?
➤ How does my DVD collection match up?
➤ Have I said too much about myself on Facebook?
➤ Are we responsible for poverty in Africa?
➤ Are humans born evil?
➤ Is climate change going to make us all extinct?

Developmental changes occurring in adolescence

Having an awareness of normal adolescent development is essential to understanding the challenges faced by adolescents and their families; it also provides a framework within which to assess and provide help. Adolescent development includes biological, cognitive and psychosocial changes. There is considerable variability in the onset, duration and intensity of the changes experienced.

Biological

Adolescence is a period of substantial physical growth and change, which usually begins in girls around the age of 11 years and boys at about 13 years, although the hormone changes responsible start some years earlier, with associated changes in mood, activity levels and physical growth.

For **boys** there are changes in co-ordination, physical size and strength. Muscles become stronger, shoulders wider and limbs heavier. Facial characteristics may become more characteristically male and facial, body and pubic hair develop. Voice changes become apparent with the voice deepening. Sexual dreams and ejaculation begin.

For **girls** there is also a growth spurt, starting a few years earlier, and bodily changes include breast development, later widening of the hips and the onset of menstruation. Body hair, particularly on the legs, becomes more noticeable and pubic hair develops. There may also be some voice changes.

For **both genders** there are also changes in the texture of head hair, and skin becomes more oily and prone to spots and acne. Adolescents require more sleep than younger children: this is probably related to all the physical changes and the linked surge in growth hormone, which is released during sleep.

Cognitive

During this time there are significant advances in an adolescent's cognitive development. This is what Piaget termed the development of '*formal operational thinking*', beginning around the age of 12 years.[4] This includes the following components:

➤ *abstract thinking*: This is the ability to think about things that cannot be touched, seen or heard. It involves using internal representations of theoretical concepts; discussing topics which are intangible such as faith, beliefs or morals, and understanding complex abstract concepts such as algebra, historical processes or art movements (for example the pre-Raphaelites, impressionism or cubism)

➤ *advanced reasoning*: This is the ability to think about multiple perspectives, options and outcomes. It includes an ability to think logically and a capacity to think about things hypothetically

➤ *meta-cognition*: This is the ability to think about thinking. This entails recognition of one's own thoughts as separate from feelings, the capacity to empathise and the ability to consider how one may be perceived by others.

Psychosocial

The main goals in adolescence can be summarised as the following three:

➤ *independence*: To establish independence and autonomy
➤ *identity*: To develop one's own personal identity that should be to some extent separate from the family
➤ *intimacy*: To develop intimate emotional and sexual relationships.

Each of these goals contributes to the development of a self-identity which is both influenced by the socio-cultural environment and emerges in opposition to its expectations and prescribed roles. Erikson (1968) described this process of forging a stable identity as *'exploration and experimentation'*.[5] He saw the aim of this process as finding a balance between the ideal self (who I would like to be) and the self-concept (who I am).

During this time of exploration the adolescent looks outside the family into wider society. Family relationships become less important while **relationships with peers** become more important. Friendships provide opportunities to try out a variety of identities, beliefs and values. Changes in clothing, appearance, musical tastes and shared activities can help to develop a sense of belonging with like-minded individuals.

Although parents may wish it were not, **risk taking** is an essential part of this identity development, and may include experimentation with drugs, alcohol or sexual activity. This may lead parent(s) and adolescent(s) to disagree much more than previously – as the adolescent develops values and beliefs that may not be shared with her parents. A parent may feel anxious, redundant or even rejected. Having spent 11 or 12 years putting her child first, putting in place rules and consequences, and establishing good values and beliefs, it may be difficult for any parent to accept having these now challenged, ignored or dismissed.

From the **young person's point of view**, the process of moving from dependence to independence may be confusing or even frightening – and may sometimes go into reverse. She may alternate between wanting to manage without her parents to needing the parental security and comfort she could depend upon when younger. For instance, a teenage girl may want to explore her capacity for making relationships, including her sexuality, without being fettered by her parents' demands to come in on time, and always inform them where she is – but may nevertheless need their support when her boyfriend dumps her (*see* case example in Box 4.1). Society's increasing expectations and responsibilities can be felt as a heavy weight. For example, choices relating to examination subjects at GCSE or A-level, or to the alternatives to remaining at school, can be very burdensome, not least because they can curtail future options. Some young people may wish to leave home, but this can present overwhelming practical difficulties that ideally require more rather than less emotional support.

Adolescent processes continue throughout adulthood, and some have argued that the upper age limit should be extended, for instance to 25 years or older. While we have some sympathy with this view, this book is intended to apply only to under-18s.

BOX 4.1 Case Example

Lucy, aged 16 years, has been experiencing increasing problems at school and at home. The head of pastoral care at her secondary school contacts Lucy's parents because of an increasing number of unauthorised absences and concerns about Lucy's 'attitude' towards some members of staff. There has also been a recent occasion when staff believed that Lucy and a number of fellow pupils came into school after a lunch-break under the influence of either drugs or alcohol.

Lucy's parents in turn share *their* concerns with this teacher about her increasing irritation with them whenever they ask questions about her social life or try to insist on what seems to them quite reasonable rules and boundaries. They suspect she might be using cannabis, but Lucy denies this, and has refused to go to the general practitioner with them.

Following this discussion, the school asks the community school nurse to meet with Lucy to see if offering her some support might help, and whether it might be possible to explore the extent of Lucy's substance misuse (if any). Lucy is not keen on talking to any professional, as she does not feel that she is the one with a problem, but she reluctantly agrees to meet the community school nurse once.

Lucy explains that she feels some teachers do not deserve her respect, given the way they speak to her. She feels that these teachers are being too strict – like her parents – which she resents. Lucy admits that she has indeed been smoking 'weed' socially: this is something all her friends do. She does not see it as a problem, and sees it as improving her mood rather than having any adverse effect on it. Given Lucy's refusal to meet again, the community school nurse gives her some leaflets on cannabis use and contact details of the local young person's alcohol and drug advisory service. Lucy reluctantly agrees to let the community school nurse speak to her parents, and tell them about her cannabis use, on the understanding that she will try to persuade them to ground Lucy less and be more tolerant toward her behaviour. Lucy eventually agrees that it would be reasonable of her parents to expect her to be in by 10 pm on nights before a school day, and 11 pm on other nights, as long as they don't ground her for two weeks for being five minutes late.

Having spoken to Lucy's mother over the telephone about the parents' concerns, the community school nurse visits the home at a time when both parents are in, with a similar set of leaflets on cannabis, an additional booklet on parenting adolescents and contact details for a local course on parenting teenagers. During the course of her discussion with both parents, the community school nurse says she understands how anxious and distressed both parents must be about their eldest daughter's experimentation with drugs, and how concerned they probably feel about Lucy coming to harm from this, or from staying out late so often. She goes on to explain how essential a part of normal adolescence experimentation and rebellion are, although these can be very difficult for parents, and drive a wedge between them and the young person. Both parents explain how difficult they find this whole process, as Lucy was previously an affectionate and obedient child, who was able to confide in them. Her previous grades in school have always been good.

The community school nurse explains that she is concerned that by being overly strict, Lucy's parents risk alienating Lucy, and depriving her of the opportunity to confide in them when she needs to. It is clearly going to be difficult for Lucy to stop smoking cannabis, given that all her friends do, but they might be able to come to some agreement with Lucy about when it is reasonable for her to come in each night. Using the times she has negotiated with Lucy, the community school nurse helps the parents agree on a reasonable target for coming-in times, reasonable rewards for meeting these targets and proportionate sanctions for lapses that she hopes Lucy will not find too punitive. She agrees to visit in two weeks' time to review progress.

At the two-week follow-up visit, Lucy's parents tell the community school nurse that they have been able to agree with Lucy on some coming-in times, and that the discussion about this did not become as heated as they feared. They were able to explore with Lucy what they are so concerned about, and Lucy acknowledged how worried she has made them, and seemed to appreciate that the strictness she has so resented is her parents' way of showing how much they care about her.

They continue to recount that, half-an-hour after the discussion about coming-in times, Lucy came downstairs and burst into tears with her mother over the washing-up. She blurted out what had been making her so unhappy recently: she split up with her boyfriend, with whom she had a sexual relationship for four months. Because he is aged 20 years, she tried to conceal his existence from her parents, but had now realised that all the deception, combined with the late nights, had merely pushed her apart from them, just when she most needs to confide in them. Lucy reluctantly allowed her mother to tell her father, who – after his wife had calmed him down – was able to explain to Lucy in measured tones that he is angry, but more with the boy than with Lucy, and that he realises that he has contributed to making it difficult for Lucy to confide in them.

Lucy's parents tell the community school nurse that they think they can handle the situation from now on, and that there will be no need for the community school nurse to call again.

ASSESSMENT

The way a professional relates to an 11 year old and a 17 year old will be very different – or should be. Factors other than age and developmental stage may affect the assessment, including:

➤ the potential for different aspects of development to progress at different rates
➤ systemic factors concerning parents or other involved professionals
➤ issues regarding capacity and consent (*see* Chapter 43).

The professional needs to hold in mind both the potential for rapid change and the importance of **context**: it is not enough to focus only on the individual.

Questions concerning the adolescent's biological, cognitive and psychosocial development should be included where appropriate.

Biological development

Early developing boys are often favoured over later developing boys in a range of social and sporting activities.[6] In contrast, early maturing girls are more likely to struggle with a healthy transition to adulthood,[7] and in particular may find the early attention they receive as a sexual object a challenge to cope with (such girls are at risk of early sexual experimentation or even sexual abuse). It can be helpful to find out how the adolescent perceives the physical changes she is experiencing, what she knows about these and how she found this out. Asking directly about self-care, appetite and sleep may also be useful in detecting the early signs of eating problems and low mood.

Cognitive development

A judgement regarding the adolescent's cognitive development is essential in order to have a meaningful conversation using language she can understand. The use of visual materials can be helpful regardless of age and particularly if the adolescent seems anxious about being asked direct questions: drawing a family tree together can sometimes be enough to break the ice. In relation to consent and confidentiality it is important to know if an individual has developed formal operational thinking to enable her to understand these concepts. Asking questions about the adolescent's beliefs and values may be one way of making a judgement on this; an alternative would be to generate a hypothetical situation that involves abstract concepts (*see* case example in Box 4.2).

BOX 4.2 Case Example

During the post-overdose assessment of a 15-year-old girl, Asita, the interviewer learns that her parents come from a Hindu background. He asks whether she believes in the afterlife. Asita looks blank. He clarifies his question by saying: 'What do you think happens after you die?' The answer comes back: 'Well, you're dead, aren't you?' He clarifies again: 'You mean you think that everything just stops when you die?' Asita nods. 'I suppose so.'

He continues: 'So if someone you loved asked you to join in a suicide pact so that you can be together after you die, what would you say?' Asita thinks for a bit, then says: 'That sounds loony'. He tries to elucidate by asking: 'Do you mean loony to kill yourself because someone else asks you to, or loony to think you can meet up afterwards?' Asita thinks again, for a bit longer this time, then says: 'The whole point of dying is to finish things off'.

This gives him a clue about what might have led Asita to self-harm (possibly she wanted to kill off some unbearable feelings). It also gives him some idea of Asita's level of abstract thinking. It also suggests that she might be more Westernised than she is in tune with her family's culture and religion of origin.

Psychosocial factors

Consider the *environmental context* in which the adolescent lives. This includes: the family context and composition, family beliefs and values, the adolescent's interaction with school or college, peer relationships, and recent life events. Friendships are a particularly important area to explore. Does she have friends? Does she see herself as part of a friendship group? Does she get on well with friends, or are there any difficulties? Does she have (or has she had) an intimate relationship? What does she understand about how others perceive her? This may give an indication as to whether she feels sensitive about her body image or relationships with others. It may be worth exploring the relative influence of friends and family.

Questions regarding *sexual experience* and the use of *drugs and alcohol* should be included, when judged appropriate by the professional. The median age for full sexual intercourse reported by young people aged 20 years (meaning the age when half have and half haven't) was 17 in 1991 and 16 in 1998.[8] One in three 15 year olds has *experimented* with illegal drugs, and one in six is a *regular* user of alcohol or drugs.[9] If the conversation gets this far comfortably, it is worth asking about the young person's understanding of the risks and benefits of whichever drug she is using, whether there is any link between the time pattern of usage and the time pattern of the presenting symptoms, and whether contraceptives are used during intercourse. Other issues to explore in relation to substance misuse are summarised in Box 4.3. The reason that co-morbid mental health problems may be important is that psychological post-mortem studies on completed suicides in adolescents show that the risk of dying is much higher with a combination of substance misuse, conduct disorder and depression than with any of these alone.[10]

BOX 4.3 Adolescent drug and alcohol use: when to be concerned

- **Early onset** of experimentation (it is debatable when is early and when is normal)
- **Solitary use**, rather than with a group of peers
- A **family history** of substance misuse
- Use as a form of **self-medication**, for instance to deal with anxiety, loneliness, low mood or traumatic memories
- The presence of **comorbid mental health problems** such as ADHD, conduct disorder, depression or suicidal intent
- Involvement in **criminal activity** to pay for drugs or alcohol
- **Impairment** such as:
  - being irritable in the morning or having fluctuating mood
  - arriving at school late or not at all
  - not concentrating on school work
  - failing to keep up with old friends
  - self-neglect or appearing unkempt
  - other changes in behaviour
  - loss of weight.

Engagement

The **engagement** of any client is essential to achieving an adequate assessment: being able to work together with the young person and help her feel you are both on the same side. The same applies to families: ideally each member should feel you understand and are able to represent her point of view (defined as *neutrality*: *see* Chapter 8 on Family Issues). A non-judgemental, genuine, open and honest approach is likely to be the most successful. Being non-judgemental means trying to be respectful of the young person's views and actions; it does not mean you have to accept everything the young person believes or does: you can acknowledge the illegality, for instance, of not going to school or driving a vehicle without the owner's consent; and the inadvisability of carrying a knife or threatening someone with it. Active, empathic listening will be more useful than a predetermined sequence of questions, but preferably without too many silences. Active listening means not just ensuring that you take in what the young person says, but also repeating or reflecting it to ensure you have understood it rightly. This helps the young person appreciate that you are trying to understand her, serves as a way of checking you have understood rightly, and also checks whether she can understand you. It may be worth reminding yourself to focus not only on the *content* of what she has said, but also on the *emotion* she has expressed.[11] Expect to feel de-skilled at times – but there will also be times when the young person experiences empathy.[12]

Ambivalent consent: The adolescent is sometimes brought rather than coming of her own accord. This means that she may not know why she is seeing you, or may be resentful at being 'forced' to come (in reality, she could refuse to come if she really does not want to).

Alternatively, she may have made an informed decision to see you, but it may have taken a considerable time for her to pluck up the courage to do so. Engagement may be easier if you offer to see her on her own at an early stage, preferably before seeing her parents. Explain, if necessary, that you would like to hear how things are from her point of view, and ask the parents to wait outside. If she refuses to see you on her own, do not insist, but leave this till later, or to another occasion. If she agrees, ask her whose idea it was for her to come, and what it was they were worried about. Acknowledge if appropriate that she is there under protest, or that it must have been difficult for her to come.

Some adolescents respond by **clamming up** or providing a string of 'I don't know's or shrugs of the shoulders. Sometimes you can use non-verbal responses as a sufficient answer to your questions, and play guessing games in the absence of much conversation. Alternatively, try changing tack and asking simple closed questions on neutral topics, such as the latest football scores, to re-establish the flow of conversation (but beware of getting into a conversation about topics such as computer games or music about which you are likely to know far less than your client does). A useful conversation-starter is to draw a family tree. If you move round so as to be sitting almost next to the adolescent, she is more likely to get involved in this. You can then start asking more open questions, such as 'Who in the family do you get on best with?', 'Who cares most about you?' or 'Who are you most similar to?' Once conversation is started, you can edge towards a hot topic or back away from it according to how much clamming up it evokes.

As adolescents are developing their identity, they may be sensitive as to how they feel others perceive them. Imagine **what you might mean** to the young person. She may have been led to expect that, because you are an authority figure, you will tell her off; or because you are a mental health professional, you will confirm that she is mad. It is important to find some way of understanding her point of view, while still if possible showing some respect for the parental (or other adult's) perspective. For instance, you might say:

➤ 'what do you think your parents might be concerned about if you come back late at night?' This may help her see that parental strictness is not just about being unfair, but also about caring

➤ 'do you think your mum and dad are right to worry about you not eating enough?' This tests whether the young person has distorted attitudes to others' perceptions

➤ 'do you think your parents understand that the reason you are so irritable with them is because you are so low at the moment?' Irritability is a common presenting feature of depression that is often described by parents as 'attitude', and taken as a personal affront, rather than a reflection of the pressures the young person may be dealing with

➤ 'it's difficult for a teacher to ignore you if you swear at him in front of the whole class.' This acknowledges the teacher's perspective

➤ 'if you retaliate when someone else in your class winds you up, you will be the one who gets into trouble, so the teachers may not realise it is really the other person's fault.' This acknowledges both perspectives

➤ 'you know the police get very worried if you do something that could harm someone else.' This frames the police as caring rather than just punitive (in relation for instance to fire-setting, carrying a knife or taking a car without the owner's consent).

Be careful of **self-disclosure**, which can easily sound patronising or irrelevant to an adolescent who may see little connection between herself and you, particularly with a large age gap. 'I remember when I was your age ...' is best avoided. Sometimes it may help to say one of your children also liked 'Warhammer' or has tried to explain to you the latest role-playing console game, just to show you are human. If you are young enough for the adolescent to feel you may actually remember what it was like being her age, engagement is likely to be easier, but self-disclosure may be more tempting, though potentially more dangerous: she may think you are revealing too much, trying too hard to be her friend, or being unprofessional. Occasionally, recalling an experience with a similar client or clients may help, as long as there are nowhere near enough details to be identifying – or you could make up a client that may actually be yourself.

BOX 4.4 Case Example

A 15-year-old girl reveals in a follow-up session that she is planning to steal her father's shotgun from his locked cabinet in order to shoot herself: she has discovered where he keeps the key.

You have no choice but to tell her father, but you need to find a way of getting her permission if possible.

It is important to address ***confidentiality*** at some stage, particularly in the individual interview, if there is one. Some professionals prefer to address this issue in depth at the beginning of the individual interview, by promising that nothing will be shared without the young person's consent. Depending on how this promise is phrased, it may have to be broken if abuse of some sort is disclosed – which means explaining that there are exceptions – which can be a complicated thing to explain before you have even established engagement. If you do end up breaking the confidence you have established, it is essential that you explain to the young person why you have to do this. Breaking confidentiality can be very damaging if it is perceived as a betrayal of trust, so it is essential to handle it carefully, or it can poison the young person's attitude to helping professionals for the rest of her life (*see* the case example in Box 4.5 on below).

BOX 4.5 Case Example

A 15-year-old girl reveals during a routine interview that her father has been hitting her younger half-brother. She asks the interviewer not to tell anyone.

After their meeting, the professional discusses with her supervisor what to do with this information. The advice is that it must be shared with social services without delay. Unfortunately, the interviewer has omitted to take down any contact details additional to the girl's address, so gives this rather vague information about her half-brother to social services without waiting for the next appointment in two weeks' time.

Two days before the planned appointment, the professional's secretary gets an irate phone call from the girl, saying that her father is furious with her about a phone call from social services. She refuses to come to any further appointments.

If you have seen the young person first, as is preferable, you may need to negotiate **who else you will talk to** and how this is done. No assessment is complete without meeting or at least speaking to a parent, but it may be important to discuss how this will take place. Does the young person want to join you with her parent(s) or wait outside? Would it be all right to phone a form tutor or head of year? Could you have her permission to contact other involved professionals? What would be all right to share in all these conversations and what does the young person want you not to share? Sometimes it is enough to keep one minor piece of information secret as a token of trust; more often the young person will have something important that she doesn't want shared – which she may not yet have told you. If you can agree on something that you will definitely not tell her parents or anyone else (such as smoking cannabis or sexual activity), this may encourage the young person to confide in you more next time (or others in the future).

We are generally taught that any disclosure of abuse should be shared with Social Care at once, but there may be situations when you suspect that there may be more that the young person *could* disclose, and you would like to improve your engagement with her before telling others. Disclosures about self-harm may also create a **dilemma**. Cutting without other self-harm can usually be kept secret, but a past overdose or any current suicidal intent may need to be shared, especially of you think the young person's life may be at risk (as in the shotgun example in Box 4.4 above). Sometimes, you may get the impression that confidentiality is more important than the risk of the young person self-harming again: this can be a fine judgement. With such dilemmas, you may need to find a way of discussing the issue with a colleague before deciding what you should share with others; but make sure you have an opportunity to inform the young person what you are going to share with whom – and what makes this breach of confidentiality essential – before you do so. You could say, for instance, 'I need to think about this before I decide whether to tell someone else about it; how can I contact you to let you know what I have decided?' A telephone or e-mail discussion, or even a text exchange, may then be enough, rather than waiting for the next appointment. You may also need to be open about needing to discuss the dilemma with an experienced member of your team in order to decide whether to share the information with another agency. (*See also* Chapter 43 on Consent, Competence, Capacity and Confidentiality.)

BOX 4.6 Alarm Bells in the assessment of an adolescent

Sudden changes in mood and behaviour – particularly if out of character
Significant changes in dietary habits
A significant change in sleep pattern
Physical aggression towards family members
Money seems to disappear (or appear)
Being secretive about friendships and communications with peers
Spending significant periods of time in isolation
Being sucked into potentially addictive behaviours such as drug use, Internet use or console gaming

Management

Any management plan – just like the assessment – must be embedded within a development perspective, meaning that it needs to take account of the developmental level of the young person. For instance, parents are more likely to be involved in any plan for a 12 year old than in a treatment package for a 17 year old. Even if parents are involved in the older adolescent's treatment package, it is important to respect the developing struggle for independence, so the young person herself should be central to the decision-making process about what is best for her. Agreeing to take a collaborative stance together to solve the problem will help the young person understand that she has an important role to play in helping herself and that you (and ideally also her parents) will assist with this.

BOX 4.7 Case Example

Serena, aged 15 years, is getting into increasingly frequent and acrimonious arguments with her parents about many aspects of her life – in particular her adherence
to her treatment for diabetes. Staff at the diabetic clinic are aware that, for several
months, Serena has not been keeping a diary of her food intake nor doing any fin-
ger-prick tests to measure her blood sugars. The diabetic nursing sister repeatedly
outlines the need for monitoring, and Serena's parents repeatedly express understandable anxiety that Serena is putting her health at risk.

Eventually, Serena's parents ask the diabetic nursing sister to arrange 'therapy'
for Serena. They explain that they cannot understand what makes it so difficult for
her to record her blood sugars and dietary intake, particularly in view of how much
effort everyone else seems to have put in to make things easier for Serena. They
hope that 'therapy' will uncover what underlies this cussedness and help Serena to
comply. They admit how powerless they feel, and how scared they are for Serena's
future.

The diabetic nursing sister is able to reassure Serena's parents that such rebellious behaviour is common in teenagers, partly due to the developmental need
to strive for independence. Together they discuss how they might be able to give
Serena more of a sense of control over her treatment plan, so that she becomes
more collaborative. The nurse suggests this may need to be combined with giving
Serena more say in other aspects of her life – such as her choice of clothes, friends
and out-of-school activities. Her parents agree to think about this.

The diabetic nursing sister then begins to see Serena alone for her clinic appointments, with her parents joining only at the end. Serena is then able to control what
information will be shared with her parents and which issues she would like their
help with. For instance, Serena very much wants to stay for a sleepover with a female
friend, but her mother is concerned that she might go hypoglycaemic in the night or
in some other way get into trouble with her diabetes – and the friend's mother would
not know what to do. The diabetic nursing sister explains to Serena that her parents
are struggling with her need for increasing independence, the more so because of
her diabetes, and that she needs to give them time to adjust. It seems they are so
concerned about her diabetes making her ill that they have tried to restrict her liberty
excessively, in order to keep her safe. She agrees with Serena that they will use the
shared time with her parents to negotiate some extra freedoms and independent
choices.

Very gradually, Serena's parents allow her to do more of the things she wants,
although it takes a while for them to feel comfortable with her going out on her own
to meet friends and having meals away from home. Serena is able to take more
responsibility for keeping herself safe, resulting in less conflict at home. Serena realises that she can eat when she wants, on a four times daily insulin regime, providing
she adjusts the dose of short-acting insulin given before each meal according to the
expected carbohydrate content of the meal and her blood glucose. The diabetes
sister supports her in this, and ensures that Serena becomes an expert in her own
disease. Although she still finds it difficult to measure her blood sugar more than

once a day, Serena does this at a variable time so as to give the maximum information, and starts to record a typical school day's food intake once each week and her eating pattern for both weekend days.

Serena's parents remain anxious about her diabetic control, but are pleased that she seems more aware of when her blood sugar is going low or high, and is at last becoming interested in adjusting her own insulin dosage. Despite their misgivings, they agree to the freedoms negotiated at the end of each clinic, and are pleasantly surprised to see that Serena becomes much happier and more congenial to live with, and begins to be more responsible in other areas of her life, such as her year 10 coursework and getting home on time in the evenings. They began to sympathise more with how difficult it has been for Serena to accept her life-long illness.

Serena's diabetic control significantly improves.

One of the simplest interventions is *psychoeducation* – meaning simply explaining things to the adolescent and her parents. You can find support for your explanation from the understanding of adolescent development outlined in this chapter, and from a variety of web-based information, some of which is referenced in the resources section below. Find out what the adolescent knows or thinks about her problem. An adolescent may have an almost complete lack of knowledge about her presenting condition, or may already have found out a lot about it. How did she acquire this information? Was it from parents, siblings, friends, teachers, other adults, television, magazines, the Internet or some other source? Information from any of these sources can be extremely helpful, but may alternately be inaccurate, misleading or even potentially dangerous – extreme examples being websites that encourage food restriction or give tips on how to ensure your suicide is successful. It is worth finding out which websites or chat rooms she frequents. It may then be easier to introduce some balance by discussing the helpful and unhelpful parts of what she has already found out and providing fresh sources of reliable information.

Individual work with the adolescent may take a variety of forms. Practical advice may be sufficient in some cases. Others may require something with more stimulus to insight or self-reflection: the simplest form of this is non-directive listening, but often some prompts to the young person to think about herself or others differently can be very helpful. Some may benefit from a structured approach such as cognitive-behavioural therapy or interpersonal therapy, which may require referral to a specialist service.

Although it is important for an adolescent to feel you are prioritising her point of view as well as her needs, it is essential to consider the views and needs of close family members also, and work towards enrolling their help. Even if you see only the adolescent herself, and even if she presents herself as autonomous, you can ask questions with an embedded family perspective, such as:

'If your mum were here today what would she say about what you have told me?'

'Who else in the family is most affected by what is happening to you?'

'Who do you think would be the best person in your family to help with all this?'

In general it is best to work towards **involving family members** in whatever management package you can arrange. Not only will it be helpful to have their perspective, but also it may be invaluable to enlist their support for the young person *and* for the professional network. It is of course essential to ask for the adolescent's consent to your contacting her family. There are rare occasions when you may have to override a lack of consent, such as when her life is at risk; conversely, there are rare occasions when you may decide it would be unsafe to make contact with parents, such as in situations of domestic violence or abuse. Usually, this would lead to the involvement of other agencies – such as social services or police – who *would* contact a parent, but an older adolescent (if over 16 years or possibly even if Gillick competent) can prevent you from contacting agencies (providing no other children are obviously at risk).

Any work with parents should encourage understanding of the adolescent's *developmental dilemmas* such as:

➤ the need to rebel clashing with the need to repay trust
➤ the need for support clashing with the need to be autonomous
➤ the need to follow the lead of peers clashing with the need to follow parental advice
➤ the need to take risks clashing with the need to show responsibility
➤ the need to experiment clashing with the need to keep safe.

Sometimes these dilemmas are not easily resolved, and parents may need continuing professional support for a prolonged period until some resolution emerges. Some parents may find it helpful to attend a group for parents of adolescents, if available: this will help them realise the issues they have in common with other families and learn from others' experience.

Work with other professionals may also be an important component of management with adolescents, especially those with complex difficulties. This may involve merely requesting the advice of colleagues: it may be reassuring for the adolescent to know that you are taking their difficulties seriously and as a consequence need some thinking time or consultation with others. It is best practice to ask the young person (and/or parents) before doing this. Given that most adolescents have some capacity for reflection, they may be more forgiving of a lack of knowledge or experience than younger children who may view adults as infallible! When other professionals have direct involvement with the young person or family, some form of professionals' meeting may be necessary, to share information and to avoid too much duplication or confusion.

REFERRAL

Complex or dangerous presentations may require referral to a specialist service (not necessarily CAMHS). Configurations of adolescent provision vary geographically, as does local referral practice, which may be reflected in a referral protocol.

Examples of presenting problems that are likely to require referral include: suspected psychotic symptoms; strong suicidal ideas; dangerous, self-harming actions; restrictive eating patterns; and suspected severe depression. Access to particular modalities of treatment, such as cognitive-behavioural therapy or family therapy, may also require referral.

BOX 4.8 Practice Points in working with adolescents

> Listen actively to both factual content and emotion; reflect or repeat what the young person has said to ensure you understand each other.
> Be respectful of the young person's perspective, while also if possible acknowledging alternative (adult) perspectives.
> Consider the adolescent's stage of biological development.
> Consider the adolescent's stage of cognitive development.
> Think of the adolescent in the context of her family, her friends and her educational (or employment) setting.
> Bear in mind the likely developmental need for risk-taking and rebellion against parental or societal values.
> Be aware of peer influences, especially in relation to drugs, alcohol and computer use.
> Be clear about confidentiality and its limits.

RESOURCES
Websites

- Young Minds – This can be a good place to start, and handouts can also be downloaded free of charge. There is a helpline for parents, 0808 802 5544, that offers confidential support for anyone worried about the emotional problems or behaviour of a child or young person. www.youngminds.org.uk
- Connexions – This is a site for young people aged 13–19 years that offers advice on education, careers, housing, money, health and relationships. It includes a variety of interactive options such as online advice, a chat-room, and telephone call-back, and even has a section for parents and carers. www.connexions-direct.com
- 'Lifecheck' is a National Health Service website launched in 2009 that enables teenagers (and other age groups) to answer questions about their health and lifestyle, and become better informed by the answers. www.teenlifecheck.co.uk
- Royal College of Psychiatrists – Available at www.rcpsych.ac.uk, this site has some publications relevant to adolescents, including the leaflet referenced below, and the 'Mental Health and Growing Up' factsheets for parents, teachers and young people (third edition 2004). www.rcpsych.ac.uk/mentalhealthinfoforall/mentalhealthandgrowingup.aspx
- The Trust for the Study of Adolescence – This produces information and books specifically about common problems in adolescence. www.tsa.uk.com
- Talk to Frank – About drugs. www.talktofrank.com (helpline: 0800 776600; e-mail: frank@talktofrank.com)
- Brook Advisory Service – This provides confidential sexual health advice for young people under the age of 25. Helpline: 0800 0185 023. www.brook.org.uk

- Child Exploitation and Online Protection (CEOP) – Visit www.ceop.police.uk. This has information about Internet safety for children, adolescents, parents and teachers. The team from this organisation have developed a user-friendly site for four years old and above. This provides a guide to Internet safety and safe surfing for young people. www.thinkuknow.co.uk
- ChildLine – Helpline: 0800 1111. www.ChildLine.org.uk
- Family Lives is a charity which offers support to anyone involved in caring for children. It provides a 24-hour helpline offering listening, support, information and guidance on all issues of concern. It also provides parent classes and workshops for parents to share ideas and learn new skills and a website containing a range of information, including leaflets on family related issues and an email support service. http://familylives.org.uk
- Relateen is available only in some areas, but counsellors from the parental separation charity may be able to help a young person who is affected by the separation of her parents. www.relate.org.uk/young-people-counselling/index.html

Books for teenagers

- Sayers J. *Boy Crazy: remembering adolescence, memories and dreams.* London: Routledge; 1998.
  This book combines examples from a qualitative study of adolescent memories and dreams with vignettes from fiction and film and insights from the author's own work as a therapist.
- Palmer P, Froehner MA. *Teen Esteem: a self-direction manual for young adults.* 3rd ed. California: Impact Publishers Inc; 2010.
  This book is for teenagers, and it aims to help them take charge of their lives.

Leaflet for parents

- Royal College of Psychiatrists. *Surviving Adolescence – a toolkit for parents.* London: Royal College of Psychiatrists; 2009. Available at: www.rcpsych.ac.uk/mentalhealthinfoforall/youngpeople/adolescence.aspx (accessed 22 March 2011).

Books for parents

- Bayard RT, Bayard J. *How to Deal with Your Acting-Up Teenager: practical self-help for desperate parents.* New York, NY: M. Evans & Company, Inc.; 1986.
  This book offers practical advice on giving teenagers responsibility, reinforcing good behaviour and standing up for your parental rights.
- Faber A, Mazlish E. *How to Talk So Kids Will Listen and Listen So Kids Will Talk (How to Help Your Child).* London: Piccadilly Press; 2001.
  This book gives parents of teenagers strategies for communicating with them.
- Waddle M. *Understanding 12–14-year-olds.* London: Jessica Kingsley; 2005.
  This book helps parents understand what their children might be feeling as they enter adolescence.

A collection of reviews for professionals

- Viner R, editor. *ABC of Adolescence.* Oxford: Wiley-Blackwell; 2005.
  This was originally a series of 12 articles published in the British Medical Journal in 2005 covering a whole range of issues to do with adolescents, including consent, health and illness, sexual health, chronic illness and disability, substance misuse, self-harm, suicide, fatigue and somatic symptoms.

REFERENCES

1 UNICEF. *An overview of child well-being in rich countries: a comprehensive assessment of the lives and well-being of children and adolescents in the economically advanced nations.* Innocenti Research Centre Report Card 7. Florence: The United Nations Children's Fund; 2007.

2 Wilkinson R, Pickett K. *The Spirit Level: why more equal societies almost always do better.* London: Allen Lane; 2009.

3 Layard R, Dunn J. *A Good Childhood: searching for values in a competitive age.* London: The Children's Society and Penguin Books; 2009.

4 Piaget J. Piaget's theory. In: Mussen PH, editor. *Carmichael's Manual of Child Psychology (Volume 1).* New York, NY: Wiley; 1970.

5 Erikson E. *Identity: youth and crisis.* New York, NY: Norton; 1968.

6 Richards M, Abell SN, Peterson AC. Biological development. In: Tolan PH, Cohler BJ, editors. *Handbook of Clinical Research and Practice with Adolescents.* New York, NY: Wiley; 1993. pp. 21–44.

7 Holmbeck GN, Hill JP. Conflictive engagement, positive affect and menarche in families with seventh-grade girls. *Child Dev.* 1991 Oct; 62(5): 1030–48.

8 Layard, op. cit. p. 43.

9 Royal College of Psychiatrists, 2009, op. cit.

10 Portzky G, Audenaert K, van Heeringen K. Psychosocial and psychiatric factors associated with adolescent suicide: a case control psychological autopsy study. *Journal of Adolescence.* 2009; 32: 849–62.

11 www.medicalprotection.org/uk/education-and-events/mastering-adverse-outcomes

12 Krznaric R. *Empathy and the Art of Living.* Oxford: Blackbird; 2008.

PART 2

General issues

CHAPTER 5

Temperament

INTRODUCTION: DEFINITION OF TEMPERAMENT

Children have individual styles of behaviour that are present from birth. A child's characteristic behavioural style is not *just* the consequence of everything that happens to her after birth. These characteristics are usually referred to as the child's ***temperament***, or constitution. The term temperament describes the 'how' of behaviour, rather than the 'what', or the 'why'. For instance, siblings may be very different in the way they respond to events, despite sharing the same family environment. Part of this may be due to ordinal position: a first child will have very different developmental pressures from a middle or last child. In addition, genetic factors make a strong contribution to temperamental differences.

The concept of temperament suggests qualities that endure over time. This is only partly true. Styles of behaviour tend to be stable from early childhood into adolescence in both sexes, although behavioural style may be less stable in infancy. Temperamental differences affect the child's environment, or at least how the child responds to the environment, and how others respond to the child or adolescent. Environmental factors may affect temperament. Both directions of influence are shown in Figure 5.1.

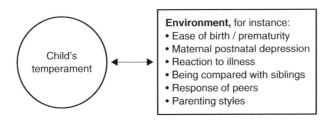

FIGURE 5.1 The reciprocal influence between temperament and environment

As shown in Figure 5.1, there is a two-way relationship between the child's temperament and how parents manage her. The temperamentally easy child is more likely to elicit positive parenting, and the temperamentally difficult child is more likely to elicit negative reactions. We have often heard parents say: 'If our second child had been born first, we wouldn't have *had* a second'. These parents can see that it is not their fault, because the first child was easy. If the difficult child comes first, parents inevitably feel they are doing things wrong – and the child's awkward nature makes it hard for them to succeed in parenting.

ASSESSMENT OF TEMPERAMENT

A simple way to enquire about temperament is to ask about the child's characteristics in infancy and toddlerhood.

How did the child respond in the first year in three areas: sleeping, feeding and crying? The temperamentally difficult infant keeps parent(s) up for much of the night, has difficulty feeding, and cries frequently, particularly in the evening and particularly for the first three months (*see* Chapter 15 on Crying and Colic). The temperamentally easy child sleeps through the night from an early age, progresses smoothly from breast or bottle to solids, and cries only when hungry or in pain – so is generally easy to manage.

The easy toddler responds to new situations with enthusiasm, finds it easy to play quietly, can fit into structures imposed by parents and makes friends easily. The difficult toddler dislikes change, overreacts, tends to whinge or grizzle, is easily frightened, won't fit into routines or parental structures and tends to be shy.

MANAGEMENT

Parents of a child with a ***difficult temperament*** may be enormously helped by professional recognition of this as a constitutional problem. Parents are liable to believe that their child's characteristics are the product of their parenting, leading to self-blame and resentment of the child. This will diminish their ability to persist with appropriate child-rearing because they see no gains and believe they are doing something wrong. They are likely to change tactics and thereby expose their child to a degree of inconsistency that can make matters worse. They are typically exposed to a barrage of advice that implicitly (or explicitly) attributes the child's difficulties to their parenting. Eventually they may take against the child and become critical or punitive in an attempt to impose their will. The child reacts to harsh handling and his feelings of being rejected with the sort of behaviour that contributes to a vicious cycle.

Professional labelling of the child as '***difficult to manage***' in his own right by virtue of nature rather than personal motive can be very helpful. The most helpful initial intervention by Tier 1 professionals in these circumstances may be to sympathise at how difficult the child is to manage. Then explain that this is a problem some children are born with, rather than immediately giving advice on handling – which would be liable to reinforce the sense of blame. Difficult temperament is a risk factor for emotional and behavioural disorder in childhood, but many children with such temperamental styles do not develop problems. Sensible parents can be told that they may have to work harder to be positive and consistent, and apply standard behavioural techniques that work much more readily with easier children (*see* Chapter 13 on Behaviour Management). A useful analogy here is that if you have an obesity gene, you have to work that much harder to be thin – but this is by no means impossible. With less sensible or less sensitive parents, there is a risk that the child will be seen as the source of all the family's difficulties. The use of the 'difficult to manage' label can backfire, and the child can become the family *scapegoat*. She becomes the person in the family who is blamed for everything, with disastrous effects on self-esteem and frustration tolerance that confirm the parents' negative expectations. Since this is likely to be one way the parents deal with feeling blamed themselves, any way of lessening their self-accusation is likely to help the child. It is also important to reflect with the family that the child is born with this temperament and not 'doing it on purpose', which some parents may read into the child's behaviour, particularly if it contributes to a stressful situation at home.

REFERRAL

Some parents will benefit from referral to a parenting or child behaviour management group, not only because of the refinement and reinforcement of their parenting skills, but also because of the support from other group members. It should not in general be necessary to refer children with temperamental difficulties to specialist CAMHS services unless these lead to emotional and behavioural difficulties that require referral in their own right. However, referral for assessment may be indicated if there is a suspicion of *organic reasons* why one child is more difficult than the others in a family: does the biological component of the biopsychosocial formulation need further assessment? Examples include speech and language difficulties, deafness, generalised learning difficulties, verbal comprehension difficulties, specific literacy difficulties, dyspraxia, ADHD and autistic spectrum disorder.

BOX 5.1 Case Example

Kyle is the result of his mother, Alice's, second pregnancy. The labour is long, the second stage is painful, and rotation forceps are used, which Alice finds unpleasant. Kyle does not breastfeed as well as her first child, a girl called Samantha. He also has considerably greater difficulty staying asleep, and wakes several times most nights during the first year. The marriage is already under some strain and Kyle's father finds his evening colic very difficult to tolerate. He experiences his wife as over-preoccupied with the children and unavailable for him. He then commences a relationship with another woman and leaves to live with her when Kyle is six months old. Alice, initially very angry, then becomes depressed.

The health visitor recognises a multitude of risk factors in the relationship between Kyle and his mother, and decides to make him one of her high priority cases. Initially, she visits fortnightly, and involves the general practitioner in managing Alice's depression.

Alice continues to find Kyle very much more difficult than Samantha. She also sees in him many of the personality traits of his father, with whom she is understandably furious. The health visitor continues her visits every month, and works with Alice on a variety of behavioural problems, such as Kyle's sleeping, his faddy eating, and his temper tantrums. She frames his being difficult as the way he was born. She develops a sufficiently close relationship with Alice to be able to discuss the extent to which Alice blames Kyle for the break-up of her marriage, her guilt at feeling this way about Kyle, and her guilt about having given birth to the child who drove his father away.

The health visitor arranges for Alice to go to a mother-and-toddler group, where Alice makes some new friends, with whom she is able to meet up socially. The health visitor also subsequently helps Alice to find an appropriate nursery for Kyle, where the staff are particularly good at developing self-confidence and social skills with young children like Kyle.

Gradually, Alice is able to re-establish communication on a practical level with Kyle's father, who is able to play a regular part in Kyle's parenting. By the time of school entry, Alice still regards Kyle as a difficult child, but feels much more confident to deal with his challenging behaviours than when he was a baby and she was depressed. The health visitor also introduces Alice to the community school nurse who will be responsible for Kyle at his primary school, so that she has a point of contact if she has any further concerns about Kyle and his behaviour.

BOX 5.2 Practice Points: how the idea of temperament can help

Acknowledging a child's difficult temperament can help parents deal with this without becoming paralysed by blame.

A child may be born difficult.

If parents allow themselves to be overwhelmed by the experience of trying to bring up a difficult child, the result may be scapegoating of the child, which is unlikely to be in her best interests.

This can be prevented.

Finding an organic explanation for the child's difficult temperament may help, but is not always possible.

CHAPTER 6

Resilience and risk

INTRODUCTION AND DEFINITIONS

Why do some children become ill, develop behaviour problems or psychological symptoms when other children in similar circumstances do not? Epidemiological studies have shown that various factors within the child, his family or social environment are important. Certain factors if present seem to protect children (and make them resilient) whereas other factors, when present, have been found to increase the chance of that child developing a behaviour problem, psychological difficulties or a psychiatric disorder. These factors can be categorised as either protective factors or risk factors.

Resilience or protective factors enhance the young person's ability to cope with life, and therefore promote emotional well-being (*see* Table 6.1).

Risk factors reduce the young person's ability to cope with life and therefore may contribute to poor mental health (*see* Table 6.2).

Resilient children may be able to withstand life-events that would for most young people be traumatic or disappointing or in some way stressful; those at risk may respond with symptoms that impair functioning or quality of life. For instance, two children in the same rail crash, neither physically injured, may respond very differently: one may be able to process the experience emotionally, either internally or by talking to family and friends; the other may have recurrent nightmares, be afraid of travelling and develop symptoms of anxiety.

ASSESSMENT

It can be very helpful to list a child's resilience and risk factors, and to include as wide a variety of factors as possible, a biopsychosocial approach is recommended. A good way of organising such thoughts is to put them in a grid. This combines the three-way categorisation of causal factors into biological, psychological and social with the four-way classification into predisposing, precipitating, perpetuating and protective (*see* Table 6.3).

Assessment needs to take into account information about the child's family, school and friendships: these are the three main areas of the child's life. Some factors may go into more than one box, but there is little point debating which is the correct box: the point of the grid is to help us think in an inclusive way about the child, his context, and what might have contributed to his current predicament.

An example of how this can be used is shown for the case example in Box 6.1.

TABLE 6.1 Examples of protective or resilience factors

Within the child	Secure attachment to at least one caregiver
	Easy temperament (from infancy)
	Average or above-average IQ
	Good communication skills*
	A positive self-image*
	A positive attitude to things in general (cup half-full)*
	An internal locus of control: believing 'It's up to me to make things happen'*
	Success in some area of life such as sports, arts, academic work*
	Ability to problem-solve and plan*
	Ability to reflect*
	A sense of humour*
	The ability to learn from experience*
Within the family	Support from parent(s):
	● emotional warmth
	● praise and other encouragement
	● authoritative discipline (as contrasted with authoritarian or permissive)
	● adequate supervision
	● a positive relationship with a same-sex role model.
	Support from other family members
	A family atmosphere in which things can be talked about and sorted out
	Encouragement of education
	High living standard
Within the wider environment	Support from friends and community
	Attending a school with:
	● high morale
	● strong academic opportunities
	● strong non-academic opportunities
	● positive policies for managing behaviour and bullying
	● positive school ethos.
	Having access to a range of leisure and social activities
	Good housing
	Religious faith

* At least some of these can be taught and learnt

TABLE 6.2 Examples of risk factors

Within the child	Learning difficulties
	Developmental delay
	Communication difficulties
	Social difficulties
	Academic failure
	Chronic illness
	Physical disability

	Neurological disability
	Difficult temperament (*see* Chapter 5 on Temperament)
	Low self-esteem
	Exposure to trauma or abuse
Within the family	Genetic predisposition to any condition with an inherited component
	Discordant family relationships
	Insecure or disorganised attachments to all family members
	Hostile and rejecting attitudes from caregivers
	Suboptimal parenting:
	• over-authoritarian or excessively punitive
	• over-critical/inadequate praise
	• lacking in clear boundaries
	• poor monitoring
	• inconsistency between or within caregivers.
Within the wider environment	Socio-economic deprivation
	Homelessness or overcrowding
	Disaster or other shared trauma
	Discrimination
	'Troublesome' peer group

TABLE 6.3 Blank four-P grid

	Biological	**Psychological**	**Social**
Predisposing (Vulnerability factors)			
Precipitating (Trigger factors)			
Perpetuating (Maintaining factors)			
Protective (Resilience)			

BOX 6.1 Case Example: constructing a grid

Amelia, aged nine years, has just started Year 6 at primary school. The school nurse asks the primary mental health worker for advice about her, as she is continually running out of school and a short distance along the road to where her home is – so that her attendance for the first four weeks of term has been less than 50%.

It emerges during their discussion that Amelia has been struggling in school for some time to keep up with reading and spelling. Teaching staff are not sure whether this might be related to her premature birth at 29 weeks. Her prematurity may also be related to her being very short for her age, which has led to her being teased. Amelia's mother suffered domestic violence from the cohabitee who moved in after Amelia's father left, and a new boyfriend has just moved in. She has also recently been in hospital for removal of her gall bladder. Amelia had difficulty separating from her mother at nursery and infant school. She currently stays alternate weekends with her father and his new family, and she very much enjoys sports, especially swimming.

Together, the school nurse and the primary mental health worker are able to construct the grid shown in Table 6.4

The content of the grid can then be used to build up a picture of the young person's predicament. Continuing in Box 6.2 with the same case example:

BOX 6.2 Case Example continued: summarising the predicament

Their discussion continues to include an understanding of Amelia as having significant separation anxiety and perhaps an insecure attachment. The premature birth may have contributed to this, and it has been worsened recently by Amelia's concern about her mother's health and her distrust of her mother's new partner, because she witnessed the domestic violence in her mother's previous relationship. Her transition to a new school year has highlighted for her the difficulties she faces in peer relationships and academic achievement. So Amelia's school attendance is affected not only by her dislike of aspects of school but also by her concern about her mother, which apparently prompts her to go home to check everything is all right. Fortunately, the journey home does not involve crossing any roads, so Amelia is safe for this short journey, although the teaching staff feel anxious that they cannot keep her under supervision. (On one occasion Amelia found her mother while out, so she came back to school.)

TABLE 6.4 Four-P grid applied to case example in Boxes 6.1 to 6.3

	Biological	Psychological	Social
Predisposing (Vulnerability factors)	Premature birth Short stature	Specific literacy difficulties	Past domestic violence
Precipitating (Trigger factors)	Mother has been in hospital with gallstones	Amelia has been teased at school: called 'midget'	Mother has a new boyfriend
Perpetuating (Maintaining factors)	Consequences of prematurity	Amelia's separation anxiety Amelia has very low self-esteem	Amelia has difficulty making close friends
Protective (Resilience)	Amelia is good at swimming and physical education	Mother is very keen to work with school staff	Amelia has regular contact with her father and his girlfriend

MANAGEMENT AND REFERRAL

Front-line interventions

Management can be targeted at any identified risk factors and build upon a child's strengths (protective factors). Several different agencies may have opportunities for promoting children's resilience.[1] ***Examples of tier 1 initiatives include***:

➤ helping an isolated mother develop contacts with other mothers who are in similar situations
➤ finding an appropriate nursery school for a vulnerable child
➤ advising parents to find after-school activities for their child
➤ encouraging a mother to talk through a stressful event with her son
➤ involving one or both parents in a local parenting behaviour management group, domestic violence support group, or abuse survivors' group
➤ involving a local organisation set up for this purpose, such as Sure Start.[2]

Box 6.3 shows how an understanding of the predicament and an appreciation of resilience factors can lead to relatively straightforward ways to improve the presenting problem.

Box 6.3 Case Example continued: using the grid to help generate management ideas

Next, the school nurse and primary mental health worker look at Amelia's protective factors. They discuss how they can build on her like of games and sports, and realise that Amelia is not enrolled in any after-school clubs, at least two of which would match with her interests. But would she actually attend these if she were not at school that day? They decide to approach Amelia's mother to discuss how she could work with teachers to encourage Amelia to be at school more, and that they would also ask mother's permission to involve father.

They next meet with mother to discuss more of the background history and share their understanding (Box 6.2 and Table 6.4). They ask her if they could meet with father and then convene a school meeting that could include both parents. Father is very keen to be involved, and a meeting at school is held in which both parents are able to contribute ideas, and the school educational psychologist attends. The teachers and educational psychologist share ideas about how to help Amelia in class, with her self-esteem, with her peer relationships and with her experience of being bullied. In this way, with a combined approach from school staff and parents, a plan for gradual reintegration into school is developed. Importantly, it is agreed how mother will deal with Amelia when she runs home, and when she can call on father for help. Mother assures those at the meeting that her own health problems are cured, and that her new boyfriend is not violent, although she accepts that it will take time for Amelia to get used to him.

As Amelia's attendance gradually improves, she begins to attend lunchtime and after-school clubs of her choice, and starts to feel more confident and make more friends.

Schools

The role of schools in promoting the emotional well-being of young people has received much attention and has led to guidance,[3,4] government-funded reports and initiatives, such as 'Targeted Mental Health in Schools' (TaMHS),[5] and other literature.[6]

Children spend a big chunk of their lives in school, and the experiences they have there play an important and formative role in their development, sense of self and self-esteem – thereby contributing significantly to risk and resilience. As mentioned in Table 6.1, the *ethos* of a school can be very important: schools can do much to foster good behaviour and attainments – even in a disadvantaged area – as shown by a longitudinal study by Michael Rutter and colleagues carried out in the early 1970's (which probably could not be carried out now, for ethical reasons).[7] This focused on 12 senior schools in inner London, looking at a variety of measures of pupils' behaviour and attainments and examining how each school influenced their children's progress, in such a way that the effects of measures at intake could be separated from the effect of what each school contributed. The findings of this study included the following.

➤ The schools differed markedly in the behaviour and attainments shown by their pupils.

➤ Although schools differed in the proportions of behaviourally difficult or low achieving pupils they *admitted*, these differences did not wholly account for the variations between schools in their pupils' *later* behaviour and attainment.

➤ Children were more likely to show good behaviour and scholarly attainment if they attended some schools and not others.

➤ The implication is that experiences within secondary schools may significantly influence children's progress.

➤ Variations between schools in different outcomes for their pupils were relatively stable over a four- to five-year time period.

➤ Schools performed similarly on all measures of outcome – in most schools different forms of success were closely connected.

➤ Differences in outcome were *not* due to physical factors such as size of school, age of buildings or space available.

➤ Differences *were* related to their characteristics as social institutions, and *were* affected by staff attitudes, values and behaviours.

➤ Outcomes were also affected by factors outside the schools' control, particularly the number of low-ability pupils admitted. The effect of this aspect of intake was most marked on subsequent delinquency and least significant on children's behaviour in the classroom.

➤ The cumulative effect of various social factors within the school was greater than any individual factor alone. These individual factors combined to create a particular ethos that became characteristic of the school as a whole.

➤ The associations between school process and outcome are causal – to an appreciable extent children's behaviour and attitudes are shaped and influenced by their experiences at school and in particular the qualities of the school as a social institution.

These conclusions were to some extent echoed in 2008 in the final report of the National CAMHS Review:[8]

> After the family, schools are the most important organisation in the lives of the vast majority of children and young people. . . . The way that a school is structured and run, and the resources that it has at its disposal, all have a significant impact on its capacity to promote mental health and psychological well-being.

There are many examples of ***initiatives within schools*** that contribute to emotional health and wellbeing, some of which may have ceased to exist by the time this book is published. These share a common aim of enhancing school promotion of well-being and can play a pivotal role in prevention and early intervention. They include the following (please note this list cannot pretend to be complete).
- ➤ There is a variety of ***government-funded*** initiatives of varying duration:
  - the National Healthy Schools Programme[9]
  - Targeted Mental Health in Schools (TaMHS)[10]
  - Social and Emotional Aspects of Learning in schools (SEAL)[11]
  - the Behaviour and Attendance Programme[12]
  - Extended Services.[13,14]
- ➤ There are ***whole-school*** approaches that can make a big difference to children:
  - an effective anti-bullying policy
  - an effective pastoral care network
  - Personal, Health, Social and Citizenship Education (PHSE or PSHE or PHSCE) lessons
  - a well-organised and adequately funded special educational needs service
  - after-school clubs, schemes and activities.
- ➤ There are specific approaches ***within schools*** such as:
  - peer counselling or mentoring schemes
  - circle of friends
  - circle time.

Other educational professionals such as educational psychologists, specialist teachers, or specialist advisory outreach services can be defined as Tier 2 and have a role in providing targeted advice on approaches that may help with a particular issue. This can be about individual children, a whole class or a whole school. The type of advice offered and interventions adopted will depend upon the individual school and the nature of the children in it, as there is much variation throughout the country. For some schools, violence may be a particular issue; for others, deprivation and poverty; whereas others have many children for whom English is their second language. A useful starting point can be an analysis of needs.[15]

The community
Within the wider community, as shown in the example above, there are many services, agencies, projects, charities, self-help groups and other organisations that are

important in terms of children's emotional well-being. Some of these are universal services available to all; others are targeted at certain groups of children or their families. There is considerable local variation in what is available, who provides it and what it is called.

Examples of *universal services* include:
➤ youth clubs
➤ holiday playschemes
➤ arts groups or projects
➤ drama groups or projects
➤ Scouts and Guides
➤ sports clubs
➤ armed forces cadets
➤ Connexions – for 13–19-year-olds.[16]

Examples of *targeted services* include:
➤ young carers' groups
➤ schemes for young offenders
➤ groups run by mental health charities such as Rethink[17] or Mind[18]
➤ the Prince's Trust programmes for young people not in education, employment or training (NEET)[19]
➤ holiday schemes for children with special needs
➤ young people's drug and alcohol services
➤ help for young people affected by parental separation, such as Relate[20]
➤ help for disabled children or excluded young people, such as Action for Children.[21]

CONCLUSION

Much teaching on mental health focuses on *risk factors*. It is also important to look into the *strengths* of children and their families: solutions to presenting problems can often be found in what the child or family is already doing, or what they are capable of doing with a little nudging.[22]

There is a variety of contexts in which this can be done. One possible first step in some areas is to complete a Common Assessment Framework, which has the benefit of pulling together information from a variety of sources about the child and his family: this may be a very useful first step in thinking about the child's needs and possible ways of addressing them.

RESOURCE

• Royal College of Psychiatrists. *When Bad Things Happen* [leaflet on resilience in series for young people]. London: Royal College of Psychiatrists; 2007. Available at: www.rcpsych.ac.uk/mentalhealthinfo/youngpeople/whenbadthingshappen.aspx (accessed 23 March 2011).

REFERENCES

1 The Mental Health Foundation. *Bright Futures: promoting children and young people's mental health.* London: Mental Health Foundation; 1999. pp. 27–41.

2 www.education.gov.uk/childrenandyoungpeople/earlylearningandchildcare

3 National Institute for Health and Clinical Excellence. *Social and emotional wellbeing in secondary education: public health guidance PH20.* London: NICE; 2009. Available at: http://guidance.nice.org.uk/PH20 (accessed 23 March 2011).

4 Department for Children, Schools and Families (DCSF). *Me and My School: preliminary Findings from the first year of the National Evaluation of Targeted Mental Health in Schools (2008–09).* London: DCSF; 2009. www.dcsf.gov.uk/everychildmatters/resources-and-practice/EP00706 (accessed 23 March 2011).

5 National Institute for Health and Clinical Excellence, op. cit.

6 Cowie H, Boardman C, Dawkins J, *et al. Emotional Health and Well-Being: a practical guide for schools.* London: Sage Publications; 2004.

7 Rutter M, Maughan B. *Fifteen Thousand Hours: secondary schools and their effects on children.* 2nd ed. London: Sage; 1994.

8 Department for Children, Schools and Families and Department of Health, UK. *Children and Young People in Mind: the final report of the National CAMHS Review.* London: DCSF and DH; 2008. p. 40. Available at: www.dh.gov.uk/en/Publicationsandstatistics/Publications/PublicationsPolicyAndGuidance/DH_090399 (accessed 23 March 2011).

9 http://home.healthyschools.gov.uk

10 DCSF, 2009, op. cit.

11 Department for Children, Schools and Families. *Social and Emotional Aspects of Learning (SEAL): improving behaviour, improving learning.* London: Department for Children, Schools and Families; 2005. Available at: http://nationalstrategies.standards.dcsf.gov.uk/primary/publications/banda/seal (accessed 23 March 2011).

12 http://nationalstrategies.standards.dcsf.gov.uk/inclusion/behaviourattendanceandseal

13 www.teachernet.gov.uk/wholeschool/extendedschools

14 www.tda.gov.uk/remodelling/extendedschools.aspx

15 Cowie, op. cit.

16 www.connexions-direct.com

17 www.rethink.org

18 www.mind.org.uk

19 www.princes-trust.org.uk

20 www.relate.org.uk/young-people-counselling/index.html

21 www.actionforchildren.org.uk

22 Thaler RH, Sunstein CR. *Nudge: improving decisions about health, wealth and happiness.* London: Penguin; 2009.

CHAPTER 7

Attachment theory[1] and looked-after children

INTRODUCTION

John Bowlby (1907–1990), child psychiatrist and psychoanalyst, was the first to describe the importance of attachment in human development. His interest in ethology (the study of animal behaviour) led to his theory that human children, like young animals, have a need for a figure who provides a source of safety, comfort and protection. A *child's attachment behaviour* was defined by John Bowlby as a *biological instinct enforcing proximity-seeking behaviour to an attachment figure when the child senses or perceives threat or discomfort.*

Bowlby's early research focused on the effect of separation on young children in residential care and hospital. In the 1940s and 1950s, parental visiting was extremely restricted and sometimes forbidden in hospitals, because of the belief that contact with the parents would upset the child. Bowlby and two other researchers, James and Joyce Robertson, filmed young children over periods of separation lasting a week or more, and demonstrated that the children were highly distressed by the experience. (Such research could not be done now, for ethical reasons – but equivalent research has been done by studying the emotional casualties of Romanian orphanages.) The results may seem obvious now, but they were revolutionary at the time. They observed that in lengthy separations the child went through three stages of response. Firstly, the child **protested** at the mother's absence, usually by crying. After a few days, he became withdrawn, often refusing to eat or play, and seemed to **despair**. After a few more days, **detachment** set in, so that the child began to eat and play again and appeared not to react if the mother returned. Before this stage, the child might react by clinging and being upset if his mother returned. Some of Bowlby's ideas are summarised in Box 7.1.

Attachment behaviours, such as clinging to or following the caregiver, are biologically important because the infant's survival may depend on staying close to the caregiver. They are also psychologically important, as they provide the foundation for emotional and social relating. They are apparent from about six months of age, usually reaching a peak between two and three years, and then gradually subsiding with greater maturity. Older children may show such behaviours when under stress (regression). They are more likely to occur, at any age, in the presence of illness, tiredness or anxiety. It is important to remember that such behaviours are a normal phenomenon. One way children manage their anxiety is to have a *transitional*

BOX 7.1 Major components of Bowlby's theory of attachment

Human beings have a need for attachment to specific others throughout the life cycle.
During the second half of the first year of life, specific attachment behaviours become
apparent, namely clinging to and following of the attachment figure.
Unwilling separation from an attachment figure leads to emotional distress.
This distress in young children is shown as protest, despair and detachment.
Loss of an attachment figure in adults leads to a grief reaction, with shock and anger
followed by numbness and finally acceptance and reorganisation.

object. This is a favourite blanket, cuddly toy or other object which can be used as
a substitute for the mother, and becomes emotionally invested with the same com-
forting qualities. Another normal behaviour that may be observed during a clinical interview is **stranger anxiety**, which is shyness and wariness towards strange
people, and is often associated with an increase in other attachment behaviours.

It is not possible to summarise Bowlby's entire legacy in the space available,
but two further key concepts are worthy of mention: the *secure base* and *internal
working models*.

An infant who is securely attached is more likely to be able to leave her mother
to explore the environment: the caregiver functions as a safe returning point who
can be relied on to be available when necessary. This is represented in Figure 7.1.
The extent to which a child uses her parent as a secure base, or alternatively clings
insecurely to her parent, can be observed in any clinical interview that involves
both of them. Most securely attached children will stay in close proximity to the
parent initially, then gradually explore in a wider arc as the situation feels more
familiar. The professional cannot accurately infer the attachment category from
the child's behaviour, which may be affected by a variety of other factors on the
day, such as illness, tiredness or a dislike of the professional's appearance or office,
but each observation helps to build up a picture of the child-parent relationship.

Internal working models are very important in understanding the difficulties faced by looked-after children, foster-carers and adopters. They are a form of
dynamic cognitive map that enables the child to understand and interpret attachment figures and their actions towards the child. Figure 7.2 shows this schematically. It will not usually be possible for the child to translate the map into words,

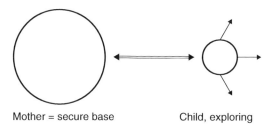

Mother = secure base   Child, exploring

FIGURE 7.1 Schematic representation of the secure base

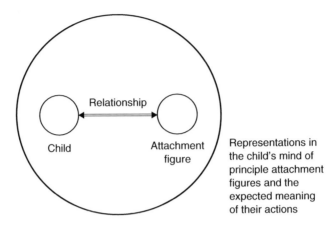

Representations in the child's mind of principle attachment figures and the expected meaning of their actions

FIGURE 7.2 Images inside the child's mind map her experience of attachment figures

and much of the map may be beneath conscious awareness. This means that if a child has developed an image of a caregiver behaving in a certain way, then subsequent caregivers will tend to be experienced in the same way, even though new maps will be constructed for the new attachments, and even though the existing maps have the capacity to be altered. So a child who has been emotionally abused or neglected may experience a very caring and sensitive foster parent as behaving in a way that she is not. Similarly, a child who has experienced a secure attachment to a sensitive caregiver will be more likely to develop harmonious relationships in adolescence and adulthood.

This concept can also be applied to adults, and may be relevant to parents encountered in child mental health work. An adult's parenting style is likely to be based largely on her experience of being parented when a child. She will tend to treat any offspring in the same way as she experiences her internal parent as having treated her. She will also tend to have a similar relationship to authority figures, including doctors, nurses, psychologists, family support workers and social workers, as she had to parental authority. This may result, for instance, in lack of co-operation, overwhelming negative feelings or (at the other extreme) idealisation.

Since John Bowlby was a psychoanalyst, it is not surprising that his concept of internal working models owes something to the concept of ***transference***, as developed by Freud to understand the way the relationship between client and therapist comes to resemble the client's past relationships with major attachment figures. Transference relationships are not unique to the therapy room: they can also help to understand the relationship between looked-after child and foster or adoptive parent; and between a parent and any helping professional.

Classification of attachment

A more ethical experiment than leaving a child alone in hospital can be done with one-year-old children and their caregivers. In the Ainsworth Strange Situation the child is left alone with a stranger for three minutes, and then the nature of the behaviour on reunion with the caregiver can be categorised as either secure (about 60%), insecure (about 25%) or disorganised (about 15%). These figures are from non-clinical samples: the proportion of disorganised infants is higher in clinical samples. A variety of assessments is now available to categorise attachment at later ages. Box 7.2 and Figure 7.3 explain these categories in more detail.

BOX 7.2 Categorisation of attachment in the Ainsworth Strange Situation

Secure

The infant expresses some distress on separation, but can be easily comforted. On reunion, she seems pleased and goes close to her mother, seeking bodily comfort, which soothes her within a few minutes, so she can use her mother as a secure base from which to explore. She tends to be more harmonious and cooperative in her interaction with her mother than the other groups.

Insecure

The **insecure-avoidant** infant tends to avoid interaction with her mother at reunion, and shows little overt response to separation in the Strange Situation, but cries more and reveals more of her anxiety in home observations. Physiological measures have confirmed that emotional distress is present, even if not expressed.

The **insecure-resistant/ambivalent** infant reveals immediate distress in response to separation. In response to reunion, she mixes clinginess with angry resistance to contact or interaction.

The difference between these two categories can be seen as *suppression* versus *expression* of attachment behaviours, with the secure group in the middle: *see* Figure 7.3.

Disorganised

The infant does not fit consistently into any of the above categories, because of sequential or simultaneous displays of contradictory behaviours, such as attachment behaviours (contact seeking, distress or anger) with avoidant behaviours (moving away, freezing, looking dazed or fearful).

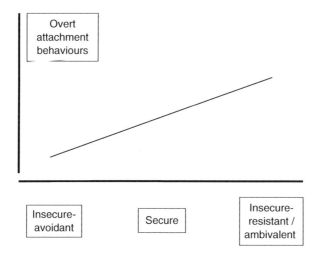

FIGURE 7.3 The three main types of attachment relationship

An alternative to this categorical model is a ***dimensional model*** in which attachment states are ever-changing strategies rather than stable attitudes, and the grouping of children who don't fit into the secure or either of the insecure categories as 'disorganised' becomes unnecessary – because these children are merely alternating strategies. This has been called the 'Dynamic-Maturational Model'.[2]

The clinical relevance of attachment

Evidence has accumulated to establish secure attachment as a protective factor, insecure attachment as a moderate risk factor, and disorganised attachment as a stronger risk factor for a variety of mental health difficulties. ***Securely attached children*** have strengths in the following areas:

➤ trust in others
➤ harmony and intimacy in relationships
➤ emotional regulation
➤ self-confidence and personal efficacy
➤ self-reliance and independence
➤ resilience
➤ social and interpersonal competence with unfamiliar adults and peers
➤ empathy for and understanding of others.

Insecurely attached children are more likely to experience difficulties in relationships, and to have behavioural or emotional problems. The insecure-avoidant group are more likely to be aggressive or hostile (externalising problems). This may be because this attachment strategy involves turning away or defending from feelings and people, so that any distress is expressed externally, as behaviour rather than emotion. The insecure-ambivalent/resistant group are more likely to be anxious, withdrawn or hesitant in new situations (internalising problems). Examples are separation anxiety, social phobia or school refusal. This may be because this attachment strategy involves turning towards feelings and people (or a person's unavailability), so that distress is expressed as emotion rather than behaviour.

    Children with disorganised attachment are even more likely than the insecure-avoidant group to have aggressive behaviour, hyperactivity or oppositional defiant disorder. The antecedents of disorganised attachments are thought to be frightening or confusing parental behaviour – the attachment figure who should be a secure base is instead the source of threat or fear. A coping mechanism may develop involving disconnecting from these frightening experiences, resulting in the emotions being expressed externally instead of experienced internally.

    Attachment disorders are more extreme still in their behavioural and emotional manifestations. They are usually seen in children who have been institutionalised, severely neglected or have been looked after by multiple caregivers. Characteristic features include some or several of the following:

➤ not being able to establish a specific main attachment figure
➤ indiscriminate friendship towards strangers
➤ lack of exploration
➤ excessive clinginess

- ➤ blunted affect
- ➤ social withdrawal
- ➤ excessive vigilance (sometimes 'frozen watchfulness')
- ➤ hyper-compliance
- ➤ a mixture of simultaneous approach and avoidance
- ➤ inverted parenting (the child looks after the parent).

Figure 7.4 represents this schematically.

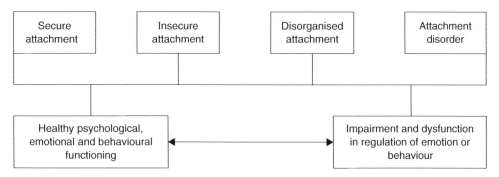

FIGURE 7.4 The spectrum of attachment functioning

When meeting a child with attachment difficulties, it is always important to consider **ADHD** (Chapter 31) or **Autistic Spectrum Disorders** (Chapter 32). These can mimic attachment difficulties, co-exist with attachment difficulties, or possibly even be caused by attachment difficulties. At any rate, in the extreme case of Romanian orphanage survivors adopted into the UK and USA, attachment problems, inattention/overactivity, quasi-autistic features and cognitive impairment were associated with institutional privation, but emotional difficulties, poor peer relationships and conduct problems were not. Nevertheless, one-fifth of children who spent the longest time in institutions showed normal functioning.[3] Emotional difficulties were also more common in this group.[4]

A new grouping has been proposed to make sense of how children and young people with complex attachment histories may present with a complex combination of other psychiatric disorders: '**Developmental Trauma Disorder**'.[5] Children exposed to a variety of forms of abuse, trauma or disruption to their care are likely to develop dysregulation in relationship to their own emotions and to other people. This may become a more useful concept than post-traumatic stress disorder or adjustment disorder (*see* Chapter 37) or attachment disorder to help our understanding and management of these children – particularly if it becomes incorporated in DSM-V. Treatment must involve a current carer in helping the young person feel safe and competent, enabling her to recognise current emotions linked to past life events, and evening out the bumps in feelings and relationships.

BOX 7.3 Case Example

Samuel, aged five years, has been living with his single grandmother, Clare, for six months. His mother is in prison for a serious crime and his father has not been involved since before Samuel's birth, so Samuel has never seen him.

Samuel begins to ask Clare more persistent questions about his mother, such as where she is and why. He is also starting to challenge Clare's authority and be verbally aggressive. At school, he has settled reasonably well, having changed schools when he moved to live with Clare.

Clare goes to Samuel's general practitioner to ask for some advice about how to deal with these questions and behaviours. The general practitioner contacts the primary mental health worker, who arranges to see Clare to discuss the situation.

They agree that Samuel needs to know more than he has already been told: that his mother is away for some time and will not be coming home soon. He probably now needs Clare to explain to him that his mother has done something naughty, so that the judge decided she had to go to prison for three years. The primary mental health worker suggests that Clare should give an honest description of the circumstances, but at a simple level that Samuel can understand, and without necessarily giving full details of the crime. Clare will however need to respond to any questions he asks. Since children take in explanations incrementally, he will probably ask to know more as he gets older. Samuel also needs to know that the long-term plan for him is to stay with his grandmother and that this is now his home. It is also probably time for Samuel to start visiting his mother in prison, which he has not done so far.

With regard to the other behaviours, the primary mental health worker discusses Samuel's need to get used to his new home and settle into new routines, as well as coming to terms with missing his mother – so it is hardly surprising if he sometimes expresses the feelings arising from all the recent changes in his life as aggression towards Clare. She encourages Clare to remain calm and use positive parenting with Samuel, as well as being firm with him, in the hope that his behaviour will settle over time. Now that she understands the origins of Samuel's behaviour and what it might be communicating, Clare has no difficulty putting this advice into practice.

Clare does not want to see the primary mental health worker again, but says she would rather see how things develop over the next few months and will visit her general practitioner again if necessary.

ASSESSMENT

It may not be possible to categorise the attachment of every child that you see, even if you had the time and training to carry out the appropriate assessments. However, you may be able to use your knowledge of families over time, and your observations of relating with the child(ren) and parent(s), to hazard a guess about whether a child is securely or insecurely attached. The history of response to separations may also give you a clue. Was the child clingy as a baby or a toddler? Are there sleeping difficulties? Were there difficulties remaining without mummy in nursery or in reception class?

Attachment disorder is relatively extreme, and mainly seen in looked-after or significantly abused children. Disorganised attachment may be more difficult to spot, but may often become apparent from the severity of the presenting behaviours, and the apparent difficulty in the relationship between parent and child.

MANAGEMENT

Evidence-based interventions for attachment difficulties include a variety of *techniques for enhancing parental sensitivity* and thereby shifting the child's main attachment strategy in the direction of security.[6] Many of the most effective of these involve videotaping interactions and feeding back to the parent about the positive aspects of the relationship. Most have a psycho-educational component. Some involve interventions carried out in the home, or in family centres, and some are carried out with groups of parents, such as the 'Circle of Security' project.

Interventions that are <u>not</u> supported by evidence include individual therapy for the child, which may be helpful, but which cannot increase parental sensitivity and so is unlikely to have a major impact on the child's attachment relationships. Holding therapy and other forms of 'attachment therapy' may be frankly dangerous.

Be aware of the attachments children or parents may make to you. This is likely to be influenced by their internal working models of attachment figures. These should not be avoided or prevented, as some professionals appear to think; nor should they be denigrated as a form of dysfunctional 'dependence'; on the contrary, such attachments are inevitable between client and professional, however short the clinical encounter, and should be used to help the work move forward.

BOX 7.4 Case Example

Daniel, aged nine years, is having difficulties at school and at home. His mother, Ruth, was depressed after his birth, but received no treatment. She was also the victim of domestic violence, and it took her two years to extricate herself from a violent relationship with Daniel's father. She has had only short-term partners since and is currently living alone with Daniel in cramped accommodation.

Daniel's class teacher, after discussing him with the school's special needs coordinator, approaches the community school nurse, who in turn asks the primary mental health worker for advice. The teachers believe Daniel's problems in school are mainly due to his relationship with his mother, which is characterised by his antagonising her when she comes to the school to pick him up, and her criticising him, often in view of other parents and children. Daniel sometimes runs away from her, with apparent disregard for traffic.

On further discussion, Daniel's class teacher reports to the community school nurse that Daniel is very behind in reading and spelling. He talks a lot in class, often answering questions with intelligence, but frequently interrupting other children. He struggles to write anything down, but can manage mathematical and computing tasks very well. He has significant problems staying in his seat in the class and staying on task – except at the computer, or when he has one-to-one help: he responds well to his classroom assistant. He finds group activities, especially school assembly, very difficult. The head teacher thinks that perhaps a child protection referral should be made or a Common Assessment Framework meeting called in light of Daniel's behaviour with his mother and the antagonism between them. The primary mental health worker suggests that she should first meet with Ruth to discuss everyone's concerns about Daniel.

Daniel and Ruth meet with the community school nurse and the primary mental health worker; the class teacher joins them for part of the meeting. Ruth reveals that she has been struggling to cope with Daniel's behaviour for some time and wants to get any support available. The primary mental health worker thinks that Daniel might have ADHD and specific learning difficulties, so the meeting agrees that she will make a referral to the local consultant community paediatrician requesting an ADHD assessment; and the community school nurse will refer Ruth to the local children's centre for support – including a parenting group and a support group for victims of domestic violence. The class teacher suggests involving a Family Link worker, but Ruth thinks she might be overwhelmed by too many people trying to help her at once, and the other professionals agree.

Daniel now has a team working around him: the community school nurse agrees to be his care coordinator. She agrees to meet with Ruth on a regular basis to review progress, and also to arrange multi-professional meetings including any new workers who become involved.

Fostering, adoption and the care system

Another form of treatment that aims to improve attachment relationships consists of changing the caregiver. The new caregivers can be members (or friends) of the extended family, foster carers or adoptive parents – or in extreme cases, the staff of children's homes, though few would now expect children's homes to improve attachment relationships. Such children may be placed by private arrangement, accommodated (placed by agreement between social services and those with parental responsibility) or on care orders granted by the family courts (meaning that social services shares parental responsibility). Adopted children cease to be the responsibility of the local authority or of their biological parents once the adoption order has taken effect, and the only people with parental responsibility are their adoptive parents.

Many local authorities and health trusts have set up 'looked-after children' teams to help such children and their parents, although the definition of which children are included varies. It enables looked-after children to have an enriched service. Ideally, such teams need to have strong links with educational services and Youth Offending Teams.

As a result of what is likely to have happened to children before they became 'looked-after', their internal working models will probably include expectations of negative forms of parenting; so it is often an uphill struggle for new carers to generate a more positive model and revise the old one. This leads in some cases to repeated placement breakdowns – this pattern further damages the child's internal models of self and other.

External consequences of these placement moves are that the child or young person may miss out on full-time education for long periods, may have frequent changes of general practitioner, and may have a variety of health problems, including mental health problems, that are undetected or untreated. Genetic factors may contribute to these, and are sometimes masked as social factors: for instance, domestic violence may be linked to antisocial personality disorder, which is more likely in adults who have had a variety of biological problems as children (*see* Chapter 30 on Disorders of Conduct). Sadly, many looked-after children become involved in criminal activity that for some results in a prison sentence.

Assessment needs to pay attention to *resilience* as well as *risk factors* – to the child's *strengths* as well as his *difficulties* (*see* Chapter 6 on Resilience and Risk). It is important to acknowledge that all children have some strengths and no child is all 'bad'. Beware of 'either/or' traps: focusing so much on the risk factors the child is labouring to overcome that the child's strengths are overlooked; or focusing on one explanation for a child's difficulties and thereby ignoring others. For example, there can be a tendency to blame all of a child's problems on his attachment difficulties, thereby ignoring a developmental disorder such as ADHD or dyspraxia. As a general rule, children who present to services for help have several explanations for their difficulties, not just one; and these are mutually reinforcing in terms of causation, rather than mutually exclusive in terms of how you think about the child and family.

BOX 7.5 Case Example

At the age of 10 years, William has been in seven foster placements and has had one failed adoption. He currently lives in a children's home. His behaviour is proving challenging, and his social worker thinks he might benefit from some form of therapy. With this in mind, a joint meeting is arranged to include William, his social worker and his key worker at the children's home. After discussion, the social worker makes a referral to specialist CAMHS for an assessment of William's behaviour.

William and his key worker and social worker meet jointly with a clinical psychologist and a clinical nurse specialist. By this time, his mainstream primary school class teacher is finding him such a disruptive influence in the classroom that, without being asked, she submits a school report to the meeting.

The social worker reveals the early care history: William's father left when he was born; his mother neglected him; he and his siblings were adopted separately (he still has yearly contact with them); and his placements have broken down partly because of his behaviour. (Another factor in some of the placement breakdowns involved younger children being placed with the same foster-carer: William could not tolerate this.)

The clinical psychologist and clinical nurse specialist think William has significantly disordered attachment and oppositional defiant disorder. There are features of ADHD in school, and the clinical nurse specialist arranges for the consultant child psychiatrist to assess William. The clinical psychologist says that she thinks individual therapy would be appropriate but that William needs to be in a stable placement for this to be of any benefit. The social worker is planning to find a specialist long-term foster place-ment and agrees to let the clinical psychologist know when this has been arranged.

The consultant child psychiatrist prescribes a trial of stimulant medication, but school reports no improvements, even after the dose is increased gradually up to the maximum William will tolerate. So this is discontinued after 12 weeks.

School problems continue into secondary school. The clinical psychologist does some psychometric assessment, which identifies specific learning difficulties. With the aid of extra special needs help in school, William narrowly avoids exclusion.

After a couple of introductions to potential foster-carers, William states that he would prefer to stay in the children's home, but with respite foster care one weekend per month. This is eventually arranged and agreed as the long-term care package for William.

The clinical psychologist then agrees to involve the clinic's child psychothera-pist. After four assessment sessions, she agrees to see William for weekly individual therapy. He initially finds it difficult to relax, feeling ashamed that he is having therapy while the other residents of the children's home, mostly there on a short-term basis, are not. After a few months, however, it becomes clear he is getting angry at breaks in his therapy and is developing an attachment to his therapist. He becomes more communicative in his sessions and also appears happier to discuss problems with his key worker when they occur. After 18 months of therapy, William and the child psychotherapist mutually agree to end the sessions.

William stays in the same children's home. By the age of 14 years, he is finding the school environment too challenging, so his social worker finds him a place at a sixth-form college that has a small unit for under-16s. Then his social worker is changed, but he and his psychologist complain, and he is allowed to have the same social worker back. He has developed good relationships with the staff at the children's home, and keeps in touch with some of the resident children who have moved on.

Management needs to be targeted at the identified risk factors and build upon a child's strengths (protective factors), as well as meeting parents' or social workers' wishes.

Examples of interventions at Tier 1 that may help promote resilience include:
➤ helping an isolated mother develop contacts with other mothers who are in similar situations
➤ involving Sure Start
➤ finding an appropriate nursery school for a vulnerable child
➤ advising parents to find after-school activities for their child
➤ referral to a parenting group and supporting attendance there
➤ referral to a domestic violence support group
➤ encouraging a mother to talk through a stressful event with her son
➤ involving other charities or voluntary organisations
➤ interventions to promote positive parenting.[7]

It may be important to think about *endings:* if and when the young person moves, consider prioritising a proper goodbye to those who have helped her, and perhaps maintaining some infrequent contact with carers she has known for some years.

There may be many professionals involved with a particular child, and coordination between the many different services can sometimes be a problem. Convening professionals' meetings and appointing a coordinator or lead professional may overcome this to some extent.

BOX 7.6 Alarm Bells with looked-after children: problems that are likely to occur in this group

Repeated foster-care breakdown

Lack of continuity in provision, for instance because new placements are outside service boundaries

Frequent changes of general practitioner

Missed routine child health surveillance (ask about hearing, teeth, eyes, immunisations, common medical conditions . . .)

Higher rates of physical and mental health problems

Failure of adequate mental health assessment (or repeated assessments but no ongoing, longer-term therapy)

Lack of full-time education

Unidentified specific or general learning difficulties

Lack of special educational needs help

Poor integration into school and local community (leading to feeling isolated, lonely or different)

Frequent changes of social worker

Association with a deviant peer group, leading to:
- involvement in criminal activity
- involvement in substance misuse
- involvement in premature sexual activity or prostitution.

RESOURCES
Books for children
- Fine A. *Flour Babies*. London: Puffin; 2001.
  A book for children aged 9–12 years, this describes a boy's experience participating in a class assignment that calls for the students to watch over flour sacks as if they were babies. He learns much about his own family life, including why his father walked out on him.
- Krementz J. *How it Feels to be Adopted*. New York, NY: Alfred A. Knopf; 1998.
  Nineteen boys and girls, aged from 8–16 years and from every social background, confide their feelings about this crucial fact.
- Waddell M, Johnson J. *Grandma's Bill*. London: Hodder Wayland; 1991.
  This book concerns tracing family life stories for children of 4–8 years old.
- Wilson J, Sharratt N. *The Story of Tracy Beaker*. London: Yearling (Corgi Juvenile); 2011.
  This novel is suitable for children of 9–12 years. Ten year old Tracy Beaker has been in foster care since she was a baby. She is sure that her mother will come for her someday. In the meantime, she is trying to rope in almost anyone into being her foster parent.

REFERENCES

1 This chapter has been updated for this second edition by making extensive use of a summary of research findings: Prior V, Glaser D. *Understanding Attachment and Attachment Disorders: theory, evidence and practice.* London and Philadelphia, PA: Jessica Kingsley Publishers; 2006.

2 Crittenden PM, Dallos R. All in the family: integrating attachment and family systems theories. *Clin Child Psychol Psychiatry.* 2009; **14**(3): 389–409.

3 Rutter ML, Kreppner JM, O'Connor TG. Specificity and heterogeneity in children's responses to profound institutional privation. *Br J Psychiatry.* 2001 Aug; **179**: 97–103.

4 Colvert E, Rutter M, Beckett C, *et al.* Emotional difficulties in early adolescence following severe early deprivation: findings from the English and Romanian adoptees study. *Dev Psychopathol.* 2008; **20**(2): 547–67.

5 van der Kolk B. Developmental trauma disorder: towards a rational diagnosis for children with complex trauma histories. *Psychiatric Annals.* 2005; **35**(5): 401–8.

6 Prior, op. cit. pp. 231–68.

7 Juffer F, Bakermans-Kranenburg MJ, van Ijzendoorn MH, editors. *Promoting Positive Parenting: an attachment-based intervention.* New York, NY and Abingdon: Taylor & Francis Group (Monographs in Parenting); 2008.

CHAPTER 8

Family issues[1]

This chapter, rather than focusing on a particular clinical problem and its management, looks at theoretical perspectives which may be helpful for understanding families – and the practical relevance of these concepts. We sketch an outline of the ways in which family therapy has developed, and then discuss the relevance of this to anyone working with children or families. The nature of the relationship a child forms with a parent, and the consequences of parental separation, are examined in separate chapters (*see* Chapter 7 on Attachment Theory and Looked-After Children and Chapter 9 on Separation, Divorce and Reconstituted Families).

INTRODUCTION

Children and adolescents are influenced not only by the attitudes and behaviour of other family members, but also exert an influence in the opposite direction on the rest of the family (an example of circular causality – *see* below). Many of the ideas in family therapy may seem rather different from ideas generally used by the helping professions. In what follows, we have tried to explain some concepts that stand out – but this does not pretend to be a complete account.

Systemic theory

Family therapy is based on the idea that *the family is a system*. Just as a human being is a collection of cells held together by mutual benefit and the need for homeostasis (keeping things stable), so a family is a collection of individuals held together by:
➤ shared attitudes, beliefs and behaviours
➤ a particular culture, which may or may not have links to religion, nationality or geography
➤ power differentials between different members
➤ its own style of problem-solving
➤ some degree of resistance to change (homoeostasis).

The idea of **homeostasis** derives from physiology: it can be considered as a helpful metaphor to explain a part of the way some families work. For example, a child's threat to a father's authority may trigger a look or counter-threat to bring the child in line, which in turn will lead to the child making a small adjustment of her behaviour, and so on.[2] The verbal and non-verbal codes that make this work as a *negative feedback loop*[3] may be quite subtle and private. Sometimes, the mechanisms set up to maintain stability through such negative feedback loops go awry, often because a change in circumstances requires a change in strategy, and the continued use of an outmoded strategy may make things worse rather than better.

BOX 8.1 Case Example

As Ayesha becomes a teenager, she finds it more difficult to accept her father's discipline. As a small girl, she was very fond of her father, and responded readily to his discipline, apparently finding it reassuring. She seemed to be so tuned in to him that she would respond even to a glance of disapproval or an appearance of tension in his shoulders. She seemed to crave his approval, and would do anything for it.

Once she turns 13, however, Ayesha starts to question her father's authority. Her mother thinks this is because of Ayesha's school friends, many of whom are from a different cultural background. Ayesha thinks her parents need to get real about what teenage girls should be allowed to do. She resents not being allowed to go out with her friends after dark, and having to stay inside until she has completed her homework. She thinks she should be allowed a mobile phone, which her parents have so far refused to buy for her. She shouts and screams at her father to try to get him to give in to her. Ayesha's father is mystified that his beloved daughter cannot understand he is only trying to protect her.

Systemic theory can equally be applied to **groups of professionals** such as: the variety of professionals who seek advice from a primary child and adolescent mental health worker (and to whom this book is addressed); the network of organisations in an integrated children's mental health service; or the various services (and therefore professionals) involved with a child who has special educational needs and who is having a child protection case conference due to concerns about parental neglect.

Social constructionism

Systemic theory has moved on to adopt the idea of social constructionism, which emphasises the influence of culture and society on shared beliefs, and includes the therapist in the system that needs to be looked at. It is based to some extent on the ideas of Ludwig Wittgenstein[4] and Michel Foucault.[5] One example is the way in which women when compared to men tend to be seen as more emotionally responsive, nurturing and non-competitive. This may be true as a generalisation for our culture, but it does not *have* to be true for all woman-man comparisons in our culture, let alone in all cultures. A second example is the 'American dream', according to which *anyone* in the United States can exploit the 'land of opportunity' to get herself an education and a career and a house and prosperity. The reality is that a significant proportion of the population is trapped in crippling poverty, with difficulty accessing adequate education, building self-respect or escaping from pervasive hopelessness: opportunities for advancement can be very hard to come by. This unfortunately affects also the UK, although it applies less to more egalitarian countries such as in Scandinavia.[6] A third example is the insidious discrimination and abuse that is part of the experience of many ethnic minorities, although the ethnic majority may try to pretend it doesn't happen. These sorts of broader issues cannot be ignored in any form of therapy or attempt at professional help.

Social constructionism can be liberating for any child mental health professional, for instance by introducing the following new ways of looking at things.

➤ Rather than focusing on what is happening to the individual who is identified as having the problem, emphasise the societal and cultural context that leads this to be defined as a problem.

➤ Meanings are jointly constructed through conversations (rather than meanings being fruits to be plucked). Meanings jointly constructed through dialogue can therefore either reinforce or challenge existing beliefs and attitudes. Depending on the clients and the context, the child mental health professional will need to strike a balance between acceptance and challenge.

➤ There are levels intermediate between the individual and the group of all humans. These include not only her family but also the network of relationships she is part of and the segment of society in which she lives (identified geographically, ethnically, culturally or otherwise). She is part of her family and part of each of her relationships; these networks each to some extent define who she is; and both the family and the network of relationships is in turn part of their segment of society.[7] Each could be considered as a part or a whole. The child mental health professional needs to shift her focus of attention between these different levels as required.[8]

➤ Clashes may occur between the family and a young person's network of relationships.

BOX 8.2 Case Example

A teenage girl who is putting personal details on Facebook finds it difficult to explain to her parents that this is now socially acceptable and she cannot see it as dangerous.

BOX 8.3 Case Example

An adolescent girl from a family of Moslem origin finds her friends' attitudes to dating boyfriends very different from her parents'.

➤ Any explanatory theory may have its place, being illuminating at times and unhelpful at others. It may not be easy for the child mental health professional to hold several perspectives in mind and use each as appropriate, but feeling free to use any appropriate model is likely to be more helpful for clients. The list of possibilities includes:
  — the medical model
  — the biopsychosocial model

  — the behavioural (social learning) model
  — the cognitive model (simply put as 'thoughts determine feelings')
  — the psychodynamic model – using psychoanalytic theory
  — the interpersonal model of attachment theory
  — systemic theory.
➤ Many professionals are taught to focus on the problems that families bring for
help: the danger of this is that everything can be seen in a negative light, including
the family's attempts to find solutions, so that family members may feel blamed or
inadequate, and responsible for becoming stuck. The discussion with the family
can become **problem-saturated**. The medical model and even the biopsychosocial model tend to exacerbate this. Many family therapy techniques are discussed below (not just the solution-focused approach) that help to get round this
perspective by questioning ingrained beliefs and attitudes that may contribute
to stuckness. The family and the professional together can develop new ways of
looking and so come to understand problems and dilemmas in a new light.

Circular causality

Linear causality can be represented by Figure 8.1:

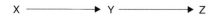

FIGURE 8.1 Linear causality

An example of this way of looking at a common child mental health problem is for
X to represent a mother's postnatal depression, Y her child's feeling of not being
emotionally held but instead being only criticised, and Z the gradual development
of preschool behaviour problems. In contrast, *circular causality* can be represented by Figure 8.2.
    An example might be a toddler whose mother is preoccupied with her own
concerns. When he behaves badly (X), she becomes angry and shouts (Y). Because
he does not get any other sort of attention, he finds this rewarding (Z). This therefore encourages him to be naughty again at the next opportunity.
    The astute reader will notice that the clinical situation could be identical in the
two examples. This illustrates that it is the *way of looking* that is important, rather
than the 'facts' – as emphasised by social constructionism. A third way of looking at the same situation could be a functional behavioural analysis: the mother's
shouting sort of attention (Y) provides positive reinforcement (Z) for the child's
bad behaviour (X), which then provokes more shouting (Y).

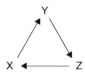

FIGURE 8.2 Circular causality

Families can be seen in terms of relationships that operate through **mutual influence**. They are composed of individuals, each of whom is in a number of two-way and three-way relationships. Each relationship is characterised by continuing, recursive patterns of interaction that are self-maintaining and mutually influencing (through reciprocal or circular causality). Each of these relationships can be conceptualized both in terms of the individual experiences of each member and also in terms of the relationship between them.

Hypotheses

As systemic theory developed, a valuable perspective evolved on any presenting symptom: that it may serve a useful **function** for the family. For example, a child's illness might serve the valuable function of drawing his arguing parents together. **Hypotheses** were originally proposed as explanatory suggestions to be generated before and between sessions with the family – then checked repeatedly during the course of getting to know a family to see whether or not they seemed to fit – to be accepted if they did and rejected or redefined if not. Hypotheses could be about the function of a symptom or any other explanation that suggests a maintaining factor; they could incorporate all sorts of ideas, including some of those described below. In Figure 8.3, the son's difficult behaviour could be seen as functioning to bring his estranged parents together. If they could be brought together more effectively to discuss how best to meet his needs, he might no longer need to behave badly. (This could be exactly the same boy as in the previous two figures.)

Boundaries and hierarchy

Boundaries were originally described as the invisible lines between different sub-systems: most importantly between parents on the one hand and their children on the other; or for instance between grandparents and parents. A well-functioning family has clear demarcations between the roles of different members and effective channels of communication. Problems may arise when, for example, a mother is closer to her child than to her partner; or when a parent is mentally or physically unwell so that an older child has to take over responsibility for the younger children, or even for looking after her parent.

The **hierarchy** in the family is the answer to the question 'Who has the power?' Ideally, this should be shared between parents who act together. Problems may arise when a child has too much power – real or perceived. An example is a child whose behaviour no one will control, or whose illness or disability governs all the family's actions.

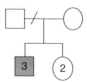

FIGURE 8.3 Family tree of a boy with behaviour problems

Life cycle challenges

Different stages of life present different challenges. It helps to have a developmental view of this to understand what different family members may be going through at different life stages (*see* Table 8.1). This can be applied to many different presenting issues, from birth to bereavement. Figure 8.4 illustrates one aspect of adolescence: the simultaneous increase of independence and decline of (the need for) parental control.

TABLE 8.1 Examples of family tasks at different life cycle stages

Stage	Examples of tasks		
Birth and infancy	Parents must make space in their relationship for a new family member	Parents must develop a new co-operative relationship to cope with child-rearing	Parents must realign with the extended family, particularly mothers-in-law
Nursery/school	Both main caregiver and child have to cope with separation	The child needs to develop social relationships with peers and non-family adults	
Adolescence	Both parents and offspring have to balance freedom and dependence*	The adolescent needs to develop a sense of identity, in opposition as well as in alignment to parents	The adolescent needs to cope with a combination of pressures: social, sexual and academic
Parental mid-life	Parents may have to cope with career changes	As they themselves change, parents may have to cope with developments in their relationship	One or both parents may have to look after an elderly relative
Leaving home	Young people have to cope with the demands of higher education or getting a job and possibly finding somewhere to live	Parents may have to cope with being alone again, along with possible changes in work-role, financial situation or health	
Cohabiting	Young people have to form a co-operative relationship between two people	Young people may have to deal together with financial needs and household tasks; and realign relationships with friends and family	Parents may become grandparents

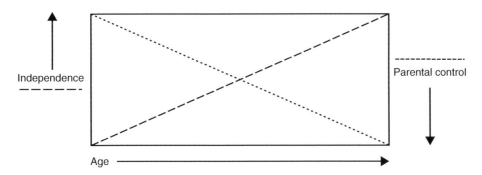

FIGURE 8.4 A diagram of the balance between freedom and dependence in adolescence

TYPES OF FAMILY THERAPY

All family therapists share certain techniques, such as drawing a **genogram** (family tree), **engaging** with the family in a variety of ways (techniques may be different for the children and the parents), and pursuing the nature of **differences** between family members. It is also important (except in cases of child abuse or domestic violence) to maintain an even-handed approach – which means trying to ensure that everyone feels heard. It may be unrealistic to aim to convince each family member that you are on her side, although this may be easier with several team members, particularly if both genders are represented.

There were originally three main schools of family therapy: **structural**, which focuses on power hierarchies and boundaries within the family; **strategic**, which focuses on setting tasks that may lead to new attitudes or actions; and **Milan systemic**, which explores beliefs and attitudes in a way that may lead to them changing. The theoretical models used as a basis for therapeutic technique continue to evolve or be combined, so that most family therapists use what they think are the best bits of each. The point of this chapter is to suggest that some of these techniques are suitable for use by child mental health professionals without family therapy training. Most systemic techniques can be used as well with an individual as with a family.

Structural family therapy

The basis of structural family therapy is the nature of family relationships in the here and now.[10] How close or distant are family members from each other? Are boundaries too weak or children too closely involved (enmeshed)? For instance, a child who has to stay at home with his anxious and overprotective mother is at risk of developing school refusal. The therapist may reinforce a relationship or boundary which needs strengthening, for instance by involving a father more in supporting the mother's authority, or setting tasks which demonstrate the authority of the parental subsystem.

Strategic family therapy

Strategic therapy involves prescribing behaviours that may seem bizarre to the family, but result in a transformation of behaviour.[11] A family may be instructed to ensure that their problem child has a tantrum at six o'clock every evening: with some families, the efforts to bring on a tantrum fail miserably (the therapist may have to disguise her satisfaction). Or a child may be told that he should try hard *not* to enjoy the next family outing, since if he *did* enjoy it, he would disappoint his family, who expect him to spoil it for them. *Paradox* can be an element of these bizarre prescriptions, usually meaning that the family or child are asked to do more rather than less of the behaviour about which they are complaining. Many child mental health professionals feel uncomfortable with these sorts of interventions. Firstly, the original strategic therapists thought it important that the rationale for intervention should be concealed from clients, but this is no longer regarded as acceptable practice, and it now appears overly paternalistic. Secondly, an intervention that encourages the symptom may at times be unethical, so has to be used with care. For instance, it is probably ethical to say to a self-cutter that she is likely to go on feeling the need to cut for some time, until she has found alternative ways to process her feelings (as described in the case example in Box 8.4); but (debatably) it may be unethical to paradox her by telling her to cut herself more because this is her way of letting everyone know how she feels.

BOX 8.4 Case Example

> A 15-year-old girl, Cynthia, has been cutting her left forearm superficially for some time without anyone being aware. One day her mother sees the scars and takes her to her general practitioner, who asks her mother to let her see Cynthia on her own.
>
> The general practitioner cannot find any indication of depression or suicidal intent. Cynthia tells her she does not know what makes her cut. She appears of average body weight and denies bingeing or vomiting. She denies being abused in any way or using drugs. Cynthia is not much more revealing about her relationships, saying she has a steady boyfriend and several girlfriends, but nevertheless likes to spend quite a bit of time on her own. Cynthia eventually admits, on direct questioning, that cutting makes her feel better and less stressed, but will not give any clues about what might be making her stressed.
>
> The general practitioner then sees Cynthia with her mother again. She explains that this sort of superficial cutting is relatively common as a way of coping with (ubiquitous) teenage anxieties and stresses, and that the local specialist CAMHS service will no longer accept referrals unless there is some associated problem, which in Cynthia's case there seems not to be. Cynthia's mother says: 'But haven't you found out what is stressing her so much?', to which the general practitioner replies that she doesn't think Cynthia is ready to talk about whatever might be bothering her yet, but she may be in the future. In the meantime, she thinks it likely Cynthia will continue to cut as a way of relieving tension, because, like many adolescents, she has discovered that this is remarkably effective. As long as Cynthia continues to limit herself to superficial cuts that heal on their own, there is no need for any medical intervention.

One strategic approach that can be helpful for any child mental health professional is to take a **one-down approach**, which involves acknowledging parents as experts on their own family micro-culture and helping family members to explain it to you. This builds on active listening while avoiding any tendency to become judgmental, which family members would soon detect and could experience as criticism or blame. The professional needs to cultivate a *respect* for the family system and of any difference from other families (whether ethnic, religious, class, cultural or other) in order to work collaboratively with the family. Family members may know what is best in their own context – this has been called the 'systemic wisdom' of the family – so it is important for the professional not to assume she knows best. This can be particularly useful when a professional from the dominant white culture is working with black or ethnic minority families, but can also be useful for professionals who are themselves from an ethnic minority, who will only occasionally meet a family from exactly the same culture. It is also helpful, for instance, to understand how parents have arrived at the strategies they have evolved to manage a challenging child, which the professional may not understand without exploration. This sort of discussion may help family members make sense of what is happening in the family, and start to think of new ways of coping, even without any suggestions or advice from the professional.

BOX 8.5 Case Example

Akhtar is 10 years old when his school asks for help from the educational psychologist with his behaviour. The educational psychologist meets with Akhtar's class teacher, sees him on his own for some assessments, then meets with both his parents at their home. He explains to them that he is puzzled as to what makes Akhtar disruptive in class and sometimes rude to his teacher, as he is only a year behind in his reading, and is otherwise managing the curriculum very well, so this wouldn't be enough to explain it. Do his parents have any explanation?

During the course of the subsequent discussion, Akhtar's parents reveal that they were both brought up in Uganda, as *their* parents emigrated there from what was then West Pakistan. In Uganda, they were members of a tight-knit community of 'coloureds' and did not mix much with other ethnic groups. Their marriage was arranged, and they decided to expand their earning opportunities in Great Britain before having a family: they now have Akhtar and his 13-year-old sister, Sharifah, who seems to have adjusted well to the local secondary school. Their father works as a postman and their mother as a cleaner at the local mosque, which they attend regularly.

Both parents are mystified about Akhtar's behaviour, and his father admits that he can get very cross with him sometimes, for bringing shame upon the family. He has asked the local imam for advice, which was to write a prayer on holy paper, dissolve the paper in holy water, and persuade Akhtar to drink it. This seems to have made him a bit easier to manage at home.

Struggling to think up any hypotheses that seem satisfactory, the educational psychologist asks about Akhtar's grandparents. Akhtar's mother reveals that her own mother has followed them to the UK, and lives with them in the same house, although she prefers not to come down when there are male visitors, and in any case speaks only Urdu. The educational psychologist asks about her relationship with the children. It emerges that she gets on very well with Sharifah, ensuring that she keeps up with her studies in Urdu and of the Koran, and also helps her as much as possible with homework: Sharifah translates. However, she does not seem to like boys, and so tends to ignore Akhtar. The educational psychologist asks: 'What does she say to Akhtar?' and notices some hesitation from both parents. Eventually it emerges that Akhtar's maternal grandmother will speak to him only if she thinks it necessary to tell him off in some way or criticise him. The educational psychologist makes no comment about this, but ensures that he has clarified in detail how differently the two children are treated.

When the educational psychologist makes a planned second home visit (again to see the parents without the children), he feels as he drives up to the house that he is not helping at all with Akhtar's school problems. He is then pleasantly surprised when Akhtar's father says that they have been thinking about what they discussed last time, and have realised how unhappy Akhtar is compared to Sharifah, who seems so successful at everything and garners so much praise. They have started to explore the things that Akhtar is good at, and have let him choose some after-school clubs to go to. Both mother and father have made a conscious effort to praise Akhtar whenever they can, and Akhtar's mother has found a way to persuade *her* mother to criticise Akhtar less.

Although there is no immediate improvement in school, the educational psychologist is able to get the class teacher to follow the parents' strategy in the classroom, by finding things Akhtar is good at and generating opportunities to praise him. The class teacher and Akhtar's father agree to meet once a week to review progress. Eventually, Akhtar seems a lot happier in school and his behaviour is less often challenging or disruptive.

Solution-focused therapy

Solution-focused therapy[12] emerged out of strategic therapy: it means looking at what has been tried that works, and what are the exceptions to the family's story of gloom, rather than focusing exclusively on everything that is wrong. For instance, parents of a child who 'always' taunts his younger sister can be asked to think of occasions when he has been kind to her, and a depressed teenager can be asked what still makes her happy. The miracle question asks:

> Suppose there is a miracle tonight while you are sleeping and the problem [you are concerned about] is solved. Since you are sleeping you do not know that a miracle has happened. What do you suppose you will notice that's different the next morning that will let you know there has been a miracle overnight?[13]

This helps engender a new freedom of thought, which can lead to possibilities no one had considered. The professional and the family together build on the family's competencies by doing more of what works, less of what doesn't, and not trying to fix everything.[14] Agreed goals can be monitored by scaling questions (rating success out of 10), which can notch up sequential small improvements.

BOX 8.6 Case Example

Daniel's parents say he *never* does what he is told: he is nine years old. His seven-year-old brother is much better behaved. The community school nurse asks them to try to remember an occasion when he *has* done what he was told. Eventually, they recall that he got his swimming things ready very quickly when a friend and his mother were waiting at the door to take him swimming. This leads on to a discussion of what Daniel enjoys doing, and how much easier he is to manage when he does things that he enjoys. These include various forms of exercise – which seem to make him better-tempered – as well as computer games – which can make him irritable if he spends too long on them. So Daniel's parents come up (after minimal prompting) with the idea of shifting the balance between sedentary and energy-intensive activities.

The community school nurse asks Daniel's parents to rate each activity on a scale of 0–10 in terms of how much it helps Daniel do what he is told: 10 if he does everything he is told and 0 if he does nothing. They meet again two weeks later to review progress. Daniel's parents rank his activities as follows:

Going to the cinema	10
Going swimming	8
Going for a bike ride with the family	7
Having a friend round to play	6
Having a tennis lesson	5
(After) playing a computer game for half an hour	4
(After) playing a computer game for an hour	2
Being left in unstructured time with his brother	1

The community school nurse discusses this list with Daniel's parents, and they agree that they can manage the situation on their own now that they have identified which situations make it easier for Daniel to relate positively to them.

Milan systemic family therapy

In Milan systemic therapy, the focus shifts to the **beliefs** held by the family, and the **meanings** they attribute to any symptom or behaviour. Changing these may change the behaviour, or their ways of dealing with it. For example, a child's tummy pain may be thought to indicate he must have something awful wrong with his insides, like his grandfather, who was eventually found to have stomach cancer too late to treat it effectively. Key techniques in this mode of family therapy include **hypothesising** (*see* above), **circular questioning** and **reframing**.[15]

Circular questioning encompasses a variety of interviewing techniques (which can be used in any discussion between a child or family and a child mental health professional).[16]

➤ One question follows another depending on the answer given rather than according to a predetermined list.

➤ The questions explore emotions: 'How does John's tummy pain affect mum?'

➤ The questions explore difference: 'What is the difference between how mum responds to John's tummy pain and how dad reacts?'

➤ This involves triadic questions – that is, involving three people, perhaps by asking one member of a family to give a view on another family member's thoughts and feelings. For instance, asking 'John's' sister: 'What do you think your father thinks is wrong with your brother?' or 'Who worries most when your brother has tummy pain?'

➤ It also involves hypothetical scenarios: 'If John's tummy pain were at its worst on Friday evening instead of Monday morning, how would that make a difference to the family?'

➤ Examples of future questions include: 'How do you think John's tummy pain will have changed in five years' time?'

➤ Questions to absent family members might be: 'What would Granny say if she were here about how you should all react to John's tummy pain?'

➤ This technique also includes questions or reflections about the different meanings attributed to the same situation by different family members.

BOX 8.7 Case Example

Phillida is aged 15, but insists on seeing the school counsellor without her parents' knowledge, and asks repeatedly for reassurances that her parents will not be informed of anything without her permission. Once she begins to trust the school counsellor, it emerges that Phillida has recently broken up with a boyfriend with whom she has been very close for over a year, and with whom she has had a pregnancy that she terminated without the knowledge of her parents (but with some confidential help from school staff). Phillida reports some depressive feelings and impulses to harm herself, which she has so far resisted. She is not suicidal.

The school counsellor tries to explore Phillida's feelings in as much depth as Phillida feels comfortable with, but decides she also needs to explore the difficulty Phillida has in sharing information with her parents. So she plans to ask some circular questions, as follows, while recognising that some of them may be quite difficult for Phillida to answer.

'How do you think your father would feel if he knew you'd been having sex?'

'How would your mother feel about your having an abortion?'

'Which of your parents would feel most disappointed at not being given an opportunity to support you during this very difficult time for you?'

'Who would be most proud of you for trying to cope with all this on your own?'

'If you had decided to have the baby, who in your family would have been most pleased?'

When Phillida answers 'No one', the school counsellor rephrases the question: 'Well, who would have been least displeased, then?'

'Is there anyone in the extended family who would really be in a position to understand how you feel?"

'If your (ex-)boyfriend were here, what do you think he would say to me to help me understand what you have been through?'

Through these questions, Phillida realises she needs to talk to her boyfriend about how they *both* feel about the abortion. Although it is difficult for both of them now they have split up, they try to become friends, and are eventually able to share some of the painful feelings involved. Phillida remains adamant that she does not want her parents to know anything, but she feels less desperate and more able to concentrate on her schoolwork. She continues to keep in touch with the school counsellor until after her GCSEs, with a decreasing frequency of appointments.

Box 8.7 shows that circular questions may not necessarily end up where you hope they will. The school counsellor hopes to be able to involve this girl's family, or at least get her to see how difficult it might be for them *not* to be involved, but the outcome is instead that the girl's ex-boyfriend turns out be a more helpful part of her network of relationships.

Reframing means phrasing things in a way which helps family members see them differently. For instance, a child who is constantly complaining of aches and pains can be described as being very in touch with his bodily sensations; and a child who stays at home rather than going to school may be described as caring a lot about his mother and not wanting to leave her alone, because he is so sensitive to her needs. *Positive connotation* goes further, in that it applies to the whole family, and acknowledges the importance of the presenting symptom as *adaptive* in some way, perhaps by holding the whole family together. Box 8.8 shows an example of a professional positively reframing a parent's efforts to meet her children's needs. Box 8.9 includes an example of positive connotation.

BOX 8.8 Case Example

Penny is a 29-year-old mother of two children under five who feels she is doing a terrible job with them. At the suggestion of her health visitor, she and the children attend a family centre, where it emerges that she expects everyone to criticise her parenting.

Her key worker sees Penny on her own to try to understand her story. Penny reveals that she has been a victim of domestic violence. She has managed to persuade the father of both children to leave, but they are still on very bad terms. He does not contribute anything financially, and she has not considered it safe to allow the children to see him. She has had some support from the local women's refuge, but has not actually needed to leave home. She is unfortunately estranged from her mother and has not seen her own father since she was 13 years old. She has a lot of support from her elder sister, who has three children of her own.

Even with this relatively small amount of information, Penny's key worker is able to congratulate Penny on how assertive she has been in putting her children's needs first, even though it has apparently left her rather isolated. She says in particular how impressed she is that Penny has managed to get rid of her violent partner without having to uproot the children; and that she has sought help from appropriate sources, such as the women's refuge, the health visitor and the family centre. Penny will have a chance to meet lots of other mothers in similar situations attending the family centre. The key worker explains that she thinks it is not at all surprising that the children are acting up, after all the things that have happened recently in their lives. Their behaviour is likely to settle as they experience more of a stable routine and start school and nursery respectively.

BOX 8.9 Case Example

Lucy, aged 12 years, comes to the attention of her school's educational welfare officer due to her increasing non-attendance at school. Prior to this, Lucy has had a very good school attendance record. She appeared to settle well into her first year of secondary school, but has not managed so well in the second year. The educational welfare officer checks with the school that there are no concerns about Lucy's academic work or her friendships. The school staff members say they are unaware of any medical concerns or difficulties at home.

The educational welfare officer then meets with Lucy and her parents to discuss her absence and also to plan a return to education. Lucy's parents seem very relieved that someone from outside the family is offering support. It very quickly becomes apparent that Lucy is not anxious about being in school but *is* anxious about leaving her mother in the mornings.

Lucy experienced one previous episode of separation anxiety from her mother when she was three years old. This was soon after her sister Katie, aged six years at the time, had a head injury in a severe road traffic accident, which kept her in hospital for six weeks, and so led to their mother having to spend significant periods of time away from home in hospital to keep Katie company. As a consequence of the accident, Katie was left with some learning difficulties (sufficient to require special schooling) and a degree of impulsive behaviour. Currently, Katie (now 16 years old) is a markedly rebellious teenager and gets into frequent battles with her parents, during which she can be volatile and aggressive. Their parents are very anxious about Katie's vulnerability and also her increasing non-compliance with rules which they put in place for her own safety. Their father admits that he has been leaving home earlier in the mornings and spending longer at work in the evenings to avoid the increased hostility at home – which he feels powerless to change.

The educational welfare officer gets the impression from this discussion that the function of Lucy's behaviour is to keep her mother safe from Katie's violence and also to have her mother all to herself after Katie has left in the morning for her work placement. Lucy manages to say that, if she leaves on time for the school bus, she feels particularly worried about how her mother will cope with getting Katie up and ready for work. The educational welfare officer, who happens to have been on a course on 'Systemic Practice in the Work Setting', positively connotes Lucy's behaviour as safeguarding the whole family from Katie's violence.

The family and the educational welfare officer then come up with a plan. Lucy's father agrees to change his working hours so he can be around in the mornings to support his wife and also on some evenings. Both agree to look into a local parenting teenagers course to get some advice on management strategies and some support from other parents facing similar issues. The educational welfare officer suggests to Lucy that her parents would be less stressed and worried in the mornings if they knew she could be happy about going to school. He emphasises that it is her parents' job rather than Lucy's to manage Katie and look after everyone. Lucy and her mother are able to have some one-to-one time during the evenings when father gets off work early while he takes Katie to visit friends.

The educational welfare officer reviews how things are progressing two weeks and four weeks later. The plan needs some fine-tuning, but is going roughly as agreed. Both parents say they did not realise how much Lucy was being affected by Katie's problems. Now that they have found a way of caring separately for Lucy and Katie, Lucy feels much more supported in her efforts to catch the school bus every morning, and her school attendance improves dramatically. The educational welfare officer agrees to remain in contact to provide further support if necessary.

Post-Milan family therapy

Family therapy has moved on from the insights of the Milan team, which were grounded in psychoanalysis, and initially applied chiefly to schizophrenia and eating disorders. Developments include the following.

➤ Instead of the team giving a single message to the family that is supposed to change the way they think about things, a discussion amongst different team members (a *reflecting team*) is held in front of the family, who can then pick and choose which ideas each identifies with.[17]

➤ The technique of *curiosity* evolved out of the attempt to be even-handed and give equal weight to the point of view of each family member (neutrality)[18] – which could be seen as an impossible task. Exploring an attitude or belief in depth can be done in a respectful and collaborative way and may also be a little challenging, not only to help the professional understand the family, but also to help family members to understand each other more deeply. The case example in Box 8.5 above shows an example of respectful curiosity from a professional who allowed the parents to come to their own conclusions about what they could do about their son's behaviour problems.

➤ *Narrative* approaches emphasise the extent to which each of us is a character in stories told about us by ourselves and others.[19] These may constrain as well as empower us. By paying attention to 'unique outcomes' – things that happen differently from what you would expect by believing the story – the child mental health professional may be able to help family members see things differently. Scripts may be *replicated* from previous generations: parents who believe their younger son takes after an uncle who went to prison may believe this is just the way he *is*, and so feel powerless to stop history repeating itself. Other parents may try to *correct* what they experienced as children by treating their own children differently: a father may for instance be very permissive with his first son, having experienced his own father as excessively authoritarian (*see also* Box 8.11 on next page). Once the scripts are discussed openly, they can be rewritten.[20]

— Ask any family member whom in the extended family Jack takes after: this can lead to a discussion of this relative and his qualities, or the parents' concerns that Jack may become too like him. There is probably a family story about this relative, which Jack may be inadvertently reliving. Of course there may be much truth in the comparison, and genetic factors may be partly responsible, but Jack now has an opportunity – partly through the conversation you are having with him and his family – to make his story unfold differently.

— A father may be concerned that his daughter is not following a socially acceptable script: perhaps she is turning into a goth or a lesbian or a nymphomaniac. He may nevertheless be willing to discuss the extent to which he should try to guard her from whatever dangers he perceives her getting into, and on the other hand the extent to which he should lovingly accept whatever she does or is. Narratives that are perceived as deviant (different from those dominant in society) may lead to social ostracism, intolerance or punishment.

BOX 8.10 Case Example

A mother who has lost a baby through very premature birth was told that she would continue to mourn the loss for about two years. When she is still grieving intensely on what would have been his third birthday, she feels she is in some way abnormal. Her health visitor tells her that she was given the wrong script by someone who was probably trying to comfort her. In fact, *some* grief never goes away. It may change, or come in waves, or become more bearable if shared or ritualised – but it is still there.

(Such an intervention can be delivered only once the client is adequately engaged and so able to tolerate the pain of something she may not want to hear.)

Family therapy and attachment theory

The danger with exploring the various different models used in systemic thinking is that we may forget the importance of emotion, not only for family members, but also for ourselves. One corrective to this trend has involved reintegrating ideas from other therapeutic models that have diverged, such as attachment theory.[21] Systemic theory provides a way of understanding the links between distress and relationships (within and external to families); an attachment perspective adds an understanding of the ways in which parents seek to protect their children and themselves, sometimes using strategies that may have worked in the past but are maladaptive in the present, as in Box 8.1. This integrative approach reintroduces emotion by encouraging the professional to stay with, accept and discuss any powerful feelings that arise during a session.[22,23] It also imports a developmental approach that allows us to see the impact of internal working models on family relationships, and gives an insight into transgenerational effects. It could be described as reintroducing psychoanalysis to family therapy by the back door.

BOX 8.11 Case Example

Christina is six years old when she is put on the Child Protection Register because her mother Jane's use of alcohol renders her care of Christina inconsistent and neglectful. After a year of monitoring and unsuccessful attempts to get Jane to engage with adult alcohol services, social services takes its concerns to court, where a Residence Order is made to Christina's father, Paul, and his new wife, Liz. Christina has had increasing contact with her father, and evidently has a good relationship with him. She has some difficulties at school but it is difficult to disentangle how much of this is due to her emotional response to her mother's intermittent availability, how much is due to her poor attendance at school, and how much is due to some possible specific learning difficulties that may be due to her mother's use of alcohol during the pregnancy.

Christina settles with her father and stepmother, but has to move schools because they live too far away from her old school, and has some difficulties adjusting in her new class. She still sees her mother one evening after school and one weekend day per week, but does not stay overnight. Her father tries very hard not to criticise Jane in front of Christina. Christina's social worker is clear from talking to her that she also is not prepared to say anything that might get her mother into trouble.

The social worker talks to father on his own, and learns that he too was not brought up by his mother: when his parents separated, he was looked after by *his* father. He describes Liz, who does not have any children of her own, as being anxious to do the best she can for Christina, but says she is struggling as Christina resents Liz acting as if she were her mother. The social worker tells Paul that she sees a lot of families that include step-parents, and it is always difficult for a step-parent to gain the trust of a child, who is likely to resent her or him trying to take over the role of the absent parent. So there is nothing unusual about this, and Liz could perhaps take comfort that this is *always* a struggle. Of course in Christina's case there are bits of the jigsaw puzzle that make it complicated, and Christina is not an easy child to manage.

She asks Paul about his experience of being parented. Paul tells her that neither his mother nor father liked him to express strong emotion, which he has come to think makes it difficult for him to know what he feels, so he wants Christina to be able to show how *she* feels, and he comforts her and hugs her whenever she seems to need it. Christina is not, however, easily able to put her feelings into words (or even actions), and sometimes Paul gets the impression that she avoids saying anything for fear of upsetting someone, especially Jane. With Liz, Christina tends to be avoidant when it appears as if she might be upset or angry. So although they are both determined to make a go of it, they are finding it quite a challenge.

The social worker reassures Paul that he has her full support, and says how much she admires him for committing so much to his daughter, and trying to make her childhood better than his own, when he is also trying to build up a relatively new adult relationship. She discusses with her manager the difficulties that Paul and Liz are having, and respite care is arranged for one weekend every four, which relieves Paul and Liz of some of the burden of caring full-time for Christina.

Functional Family Therapy[24]

Functional Family Therapy is a model of systemic psychotherapy developed in North America that has accrued an impressive evidence base since its early development in 1972.[25] It has been shown to be effective in reducing offending and other antisocial behaviours in the 10–18 year age range[26] and shows promise in reducing adolescent drug use.[27] It is now being tested as an intervention to prevent children becoming looked after and to support early return home. Cost-effectiveness (through reducing the rate of reoffending) has been established in a 'real world' setting:[28] this depends on competent therapists following the manual closely.[29] As well as being used widely in the USA, it is currently in use as part of normal service delivery in Norway, Sweden and Holland. Its initial deployment in the UK is based in Brighton, where (at the time of writing this chapter) it is the subject of a randomised controlled trial.[30]

Functional Family Therapy is an assertive outreach model that usually involves 12–16 sessions, starting very intensively and becoming less frequent. As in multisystemic therapy (*see* Chapter 30 on Disorders of Conduct), each worker's caseload is limited to about 10 families, and most of the work is done in the family's home. The model has three stages.

➤ The first stage is **engagement and motivation**, using a focus on relationships rather than individuals. Behaviours of concern are reframed as having 'noble intent', emphasising the positive aspects of the emotional bonds between family members. The therapist quickly interrupts any negativity or emerging arguments and instils hope for change. Careful attention is given to engaging the young person as well as carers, to ensure that a balanced alliance with all family members is achieved. This engagement has been shown to be crucial to the effectiveness of the intervention.

➤ The middle stage looks at possibilities for ***behaviour change***, building a plan individually tailored to the family members that includes careful attention to their relational style and is based on their strengths and protective factors. The therapist must also help the family address risk factors and develop new skills, such as better communication and problem solving, finding less conflictual ways of expressing emotion and learning how to stay out of trouble.

➤ The consolidation stage is called ***generalisation***: family members apply their newly learned skills to situations in the outside world and anticipate future situations. The therapist predicts relapse to help the family generate strategies to cope with things that are likely to go wrong. Liaison with other involved agencies is essential, and referral may be necessary to others who should be involved.

BOX 8.12 Case Example illustrating Functional Family Therapy

Background

Jane is 15 years old and lives with her mother, Jolene, and two brothers in temporary accommodation. As a result of the screaming and shouting that comes from the house, the family have been evicted five times in the past six years. Jane regularly 'trashes the house', smashing up furniture and destroying Jolene's belongings. Jane is on a youth rehabilitation order and is working with the Youth Offending Service due to two violent offences that occurred while she was under the influence of alcohol. Jane also uses cannabis regularly. She frequently leaves the house and stays out all night without Jolene knowing where she is. Jane has episodes of low mood during which she cuts her arms and legs; she has taken two overdoses. Jolene also has prolonged periods of low mood and has been prescribed antidepressants, but does not take them. She worries that she has no influence over Jane; she feels hopeless and angry and has very low self-esteem.

Jane has been excluded from one school and, although she works well in the new school when she is there, her attendance averages below 40%. She has a diagnosis of ADHD, but has never taken her medication regularly.

Engagement and motivation

The initial work with Jane and Jolene focuses on trying to reduce the intense conflict and negativity in their relationship and increase the bond between them. The therapist acknowledges the hopelessness they both feel and helps them think about the possibility that, beneath the anger they show to each other, they are both feeling sad and very hurt.

The therapist forms the view that their pattern of conflict has not only enabled them to come together in an intense way but also to achieve distance from each other. Both Jane and Jolene seem to want a degree of closeness but each needs her own space – finding a balance is difficult.

Behaviour change

The next phase of therapy focuses on helping Jane and Jolene find safer ways of communicating their need for time together and apart. The therapist also helps them both with anger management and emotional regulation skills. When they both feel more confident in their ability to stay calm, the therapist helps them practice listening and communication skills within the session.

As communication improves between them, Jane and Jolene develop strategies that enable them to negotiate and jointly engage in problem-solving when issues arise.

Generalisation

In the final phase of therapy, Jane and Jolene explore ways in which they can use their recently developed skills in novel situations. For example, Jane decides she will tell her teacher when she needs time out of the class rather than just storming out. Jolene decides she will spend time with her younger son, using some of the listening and negotiation skills she has developed with Jane.

Outcomes

The family are seen for a period of six months. After two months, as communication between Jane and Jolene improves, there is a significant reduction in complaints from neighbours, and after four months, the complaints have stopped completely.

Jane does not offend again during this time and significantly reduces her use of cannabis and alcohol. She does not engage in risky or self-harming behaviour, even during a period of low mood.

Jolene reports feeling much more confident in her relationship with both Jane and her younger son. She also decides to get a job.

RELEVANCE OF FAMILY THERAPY

Systemic family therapy has been shown to be effective in a number of settings and for a variety of different conditions. There is good evidence for its effectiveness in particular in the treatment of conduct disorders, substance misuse and eating disorders; and it probably enhances the effectiveness of other treatments for depression and chronic illness.[31] It may be necessary to tailor the type of therapy to the condition being treated, as well as the nature of the clients and their context. In a well-resourced service, family therapy can be delivered by a team, using a one-way screen. Family therapy or its various techniques can also be delivered in non-specialist settings (including at home).

The *ideas* can be used by any professional working in child mental health. For instance, it is helpful in general to develop a systemic perspective in dealing with all the families you see, and also with professional organisations – including your own. A useful question to ask yourself of any symptom in a child is: 'What *function* is this symptom serving for this family?' or the 'Balint question': 'What makes *this* child present with *this* symptom at *this* time?'[32] Another is: '*What life cycle stage is contributing to this symptom?*' The overall way-of-looking is to try to see the presenting symptom as reflecting relationships and social or cultural conflicts rather than focusing just on the individual.

BOX 8.13 Case Example

Concerns about Glen's weight, height and immaturity are raised with the community school nurse by Glen's mother, Fiona. Glen is about to move up to secondary school and his mother is becoming increasingly anxious that Glen will get bullied. She has had him investigated by a paediatrician because of his short stature, which has been attributed to familial growth delay; he also has a restricted and faddy diet. Fiona recalls that Glen has always been small for his age. As he has got older, Fiona has become increasingly anxious about his food intake, which she has begun to monitor.

The community school nurse meets with Glen on a couple of occasions to check with him whether he has any worries about his height, weight or transition to secondary school. Glen denies any worries about his height or weight, but admits to feeling irritated that his mother seems to focus so much on this. Aside from this, the community school nurse picks up that Glen *does* have some worries about moving to secondary school and also about growing up. He tells her that his two older siblings have both left home and have families of their own, each with their respective difficulties. In addition, Glen seems to spend most of his free time with his mother rather than his brothers or his father, who works long hours.

The community school nurse then meets with both Glen's parents (without him). She attempts to reframe Glen's restricted eating as an expression of his fear of growing up. She encourages Glen's father to spend some one-to-one time with Glen whenever possible, to help strengthen their relationship and to act as a positive male role-model. The community school nurse also suggests that Glen and his father look together at photos of his dad growing up, as father was also a late developer and had to cope with this at school. The community school nurse also encourages Fiona to find some interests of her own that are independent from Glen, and to try not to show how anxious she is about what he eats – as this may inadvertently exacerbate the problem.

A month later, the community school nurse meets with Fiona to check on progress. Although Glen's father has struggled to make time for some of the ideas suggested, Fiona has joined a weekly art class. While Fiona is at the art class, Glen and his father spend the evening together – either watching a film or playing computer games together; they have also found time to look at photographs of father as a child. Glen's appetite seems to have improved, perhaps because Fiona has stopped logging his daily intake. Glen has been on a trip to his new school with his class group and this seems to have reduced his anxiety about the new school.

With parents' permission, the community school nurse suggests to the new school that they should encourage Glen to join some after-school activities to help develop his friendships and separate further from his mother. She agrees to monitor how Glen gets on after he has changed schools, but otherwise makes no further appointments.

Practical applications of family therapy ideas

For any illness or problem, think about its *function* for the family, as well as its *cause*.

Think about *repeated interactional patterns*, rather than one person causing another's behaviour. For instance, a mother's behaviour to her difficult child may be as much due to the effect of his behaviour on *her* as the cause of *his* difficulties.

Does the parental subsystem need strengthening? If so, seeing both parents together may be invaluable, as with the family described in Box 8.13.

Looking for solutions rather than problems. Find out what parents have done that works: this can be very affirming for them, and may lead to the development of more solutions. It also avoids the uncomfortable situation of discussing everything a parent dislikes about the child in front of him.

Are disagreements in the family a reflection of *clashing beliefs or cultures*?

Are any family members following a *script* that they need help to rewrite?

Can you use *curiosity* in a respectful way to explore beliefs and attitudes?

Can you help a client *transform* her understanding of a presenting problem from something that is individual and perhaps to do with things going on inside her to something that has to do with her relationships with others, her family scripts or her cultural beliefs?

Try to find opportunities to *reframe things positively*, while still respecting feelings.

➤ In the family described in Box 8.1, Ayesha's father could be commended for caring so much about his daughter that he is prepared to protect her much more than other parents do. *However*, care should be taken if this is said in Ayesha's presence that it does not alienate her by making her feel the professional is taking her parents' side. Ensure she is fully engaged first, otherwise you risk losing neutrality. Alternatively, see her parents for a brief period without her.

➤ Cynthia, described in Box 8.4, could be described as protecting her parents from whatever might be bothering her.

➤ With Akhtar's parents, described in Box 8.5, the educational psychologist may be able to say, once he has got to know them well enough, that it is just as well Akhtar was showing problems in school, otherwise none of them would have realised how unhappy he was.

➤ Phillida's actions in Box 8.7 may make the school counsellor's life rather difficult – it would be so much easier for her if she were allowed to share her concerns with Phillida's parents – but Phillida could be commended for sorting out her abortion without worrying her parents, overcoming her anger with her boyfriend enough to talk with him as a friend, sharing with him her feelings about the abortion, and also listening to *his* feelings about it.

➤ Christina's social worker (Box 8.11) could say to her father how impressed she is that he is so thoughtful about his own childhood, and that he is trying to learn lessons from it so that Christina's experience of being looked after is more positive.

➤ The community school nurse could reframe the apparently overprotective attitude of Glen's mother Fiona, described in Box 8.13, as very sensible and proactive, given that she is trying to ensure he has the best possible start to secondary school and grows as well as he can.

➤ If a child wrecks the room in which you are seeing him, try saying something to his parents like: 'Well, he's being very helpful in showing me what sort of difficulties you must have with him at home.'

➤ Of a teenager who is depressed after her grandmother's death, you might say: 'She's doing a good job of showing how sad you all are.'

Emphasising some of the less blaming factors can be a great help for parents, as they may feel more able to cope with something which they can join with you to fight against. This is called *externalizing the problem*. The traditional example is to describe faecal incontinence as 'sneaky poo' – something that creeps up on you and messes you up.[33] It is important to describe the problem in terms which make it seem no one's fault. Other examples include the following.

➤ Attributing any relationship difficulties between the adolescent girls and parents mentioned in Boxes 8.1 to 8.3 to a clash of different cultures can serve to emphasise that it is no one individual's fault.

➤ Blaming Daniel's overuse of computer games, described in Box 8.6, on a cultural drift towards such screen-oriented activities may help obviate his parents' potential guilt about using a computer games console as a convenient babysitter.

➤ Penny's difficulties described in Box 8.8 could be ascribed to the high prevalence of domestic violence in our culture (or parts of it), to the power imbalance between men and women, to the difficulty for so many children who have absent fathers, or to whatever sociopolitical view Penny and her key worker can agree on.

➤ Attributing Lucy's difficulties in Box 8.9 to the awful accident that happened to her sister Katie may help her parents feel less guilty about the extent to which they temporarily ignored the needs of their healthier daughter.

➤ Describing the grief of the mother in Box 8.10 as something that comes over her and seems to overwhelm her from outside may help her realise that she is experiencing a normal reaction to an untoward event, rather than something being intrinsically wrong with *her*.

➤ The social worker could re-emphasise to Christina's father (Box 8.11) that several circumstances have come together to make Christina difficult for anyone to parent, and he and his second wife are doing a grand job.

➤ With the family described in Box 8.13, it may be worthwhile for the community school nurse to say that Fiona's maternal worries about Glen's transfer to secondary school are entirely justified, given Glen's size, since transition from primary to secondary school is a difficult challenge for many children.

➤ Blaming relationship difficulties between a mother and five-year-old child on the difficult start to life they have both had due to prematurity and postnatal depression may help them realise that their mutual conflict may not be the fault of either one of them – although this is a tricky situation, since a mother who has had postnatal depression may feel it is her fault that she was depressed and was unable to give her child enough positive attention.

➤ Attributing behaviour problems in school to specific learning difficulties rather than relationships at home, as the school has supposed, may help move things forward more effectively.

Try thinking about the power imbalances, subsystems and boundaries within your own *professional network*. This can be particularly useful when you are unsure how to handle inter-professional problems, perhaps stuck thinking that they are due to personalities.

REFERENCES

1 This chapter has been greatly improved by input from Gill Goodwillie, Lead Practitioner in Systemic Psychotherapy, Wolverhampton Primary Care Trust.

2 Goodman R, Scott S. *Child Psychiatry*. Oxford: Wiley-Blackwell; 2005.

3 Bateson G. *Steps to an Ecology of Mind: collected essays in anthropology, psychiatry, evolution and epistemology*. Chicago, IL: Chicago University Press; 2000.

4 Wittgenstein L, von Wright GH, Anscombe GEM. *On Certainty*. London: Harper Collins; 2001.

5 Foucault M. *The Archaeology of Knowledge*. London: Tavistock; 1975.

6 Wilkinson R, Pickett K. *The Spirit Level: why more equal societies almost always do better*. London: Allen Lane; 2009.

7 Pearce WB, Cronen VE. *Communication, Action and Meaning: the creation of social realities*. New York, NY: Praeger; 1980.

8 Kozlowska K, Hanney L. The network perspective: an integration of attachment and family systems theories. *Fam Process*. 2002; **41**(3): 285–312.

9 Anderson H, Goolishian Minuchin S. *Families and Family Therapy*. Boston, MA: Harvard University Press; 1974.

10 Minuchin S. *Families and Family Therapy*. Boston: Harvard University Press; 1974.

11 Haley J. *Uncommon Therapy: psychiatric techniques of Milton H Erickson, MD*. New York, NY: WW Norton; 1993.

12 De Shazer S. *Patterns of Brief Therapy: an ecosystemic approach*. New York, NY: Guilford Press; 1982.

13 Berg IM. *Family Preservation: a brief therapy workbook*. London: BT Press; 1991.

14 Dallos R, Draper R. *An Introduction to Family Therapy: systemic theory and practice*. 2nd ed. Maidenhead: Open University Press; 2005.

15 Palazzoli MS, Boscolo L, Cecchin G, *et al.* Hypothesizing – circularity – neutrality: three guidelines for the conductor of the session. *Fam Process*. 1980; **19**(1): 3–12.

16 Tomm K. Interventive interviewing, part III: intending to ask lineal, circular, strategic, or reflexive questions? *Fam Process*. 1988; **27**(1): 1–15.

17 Andersen T. The reflecting team: dialogue and meta-dialogue in clinical work. *Fam Process*. 1987; **26**(4): 415–28.

18 Cecchin G. Hypothesizing, circularity, and neutrality revisited: an invitation to curiosity. *Fam Process*. 1987; **26**(4): 405–13.

19 White M, Epston D. *Narrative Means to Therapeutic Ends*. New York, NY: WW Norton; 1990.

20 Byng-Hall J. *Rewriting Family Scripts: improvisation and systems change*. New York, NY: Guilford Press; 1996.

21 Crittenden PM, Dallos R. All in the family: integrating attachment and family systems theories. *Clinical Child Psychology & Psychiatry.* 2009; **14**(3): 389–409.

22 Gerhardt S. *Why Love Matters.* London: Routledge; 2004.

23 Dallos R, Vetere A. *Systemic Therapy and Attachment Narratives.* London: Routledge; 2009.

24 We are indebted to Moira Doolan, Consultant Systemic Psychotherapist, National Academy for Parenting Research, Institute of Psychiatry; and Joanna Pearse, Consultant Systemic Psychotherapist, Functional Family Therapist/Supervisor, Brighton and Hove Children and Young People's Trust for help in writing this section and providing the case example.

25 www.fftinc.com

26 Klein N, Alexander J, Parsons B. Impact of family systems intervention on recidivism and sibling delinquency: a model of primary prevention and program evaluation. *J Consult Clin Psychol.* 1977; **45**(3): 469–74.

27 Waldron H, Slesnick N, Brody J, *et al.* Treatment outcomes for adolescent substance abuse at 4- and 7-month assessments. *J Consult Clin Psychol.* 2001; **69**(5): 802–13.

28 Barnoski R. *Outcome Evaluation of Washington State Research-Based Programs for Juvenile Offenders.* Seattle, WA: Washington State Institute of Public Policy; 2004. Available at: www.wsipp.wa.gov/pub.asp?docid=04-01-1201 (accessed 23 March 2011).

29 Sexton T, Turner CW. The effectiveness of functional family therapy for youth with behavioral problems in a community practice setting. *J Fam Psychol.* 2010; **24**(3): 339–48.

30 Doolan M, Pearse J. *Creating Hope? Can Functional Family Therapy succeed in reducing offending in a British context?* [workshop presentation at Royal College of Psychiatrists' Faculty of Child and Adolescent Psychiatry annual meeting]. St Catherine's College, Oxford; 30 September 2010.

31 Cottrell D, Boston P. Practitioner review: the effectiveness of systemic family therapy for children and adolescents. *J Child Psychol Psychiatry.* 2002; **43**(5): 573–86.

32 Balint M. *The Doctor, His Patient and The Illness.* 2nd ed. London: Churchill Livingstone; 2000.

33 White, op. cit.

CHAPTER 9

Separation, divorce and reconstituted families

INTRODUCTION

Epidemiology

At least one in four children will experience the divorce of their parents by the time they are 16 years old.[1] Divorce figures from 2008 show that a total of 106 763 children under the age of 16 years in England and Wales experienced the divorce of their parents.[2] Of the 11.2 per 1 000 married couples who divorced, about half had children under 16, each of these couples having an average of 1.76 children living with them, including children of previous marriages, adopted and stepchildren. Of these 106 763 children, 21% were under five years old, 42% were aged 5–11 years and 37% were aged 11–15 years.

These figures do not include children who experience the separation of their unmarried parents. The number of marriages is gradually declining, as cohabitation increases: 15% of mothers who give birth are already living alone, 25% are cohabiting and 60% are married.[3] Many children become attached to a parental cohabitee. So the proportion of children experiencing separation of the adults who have been caring for them is probably considerably more than one in four. Temporary separation may also have an impact, for instance due to a parent working abroad or being in prison.

Effects of parental separation on children

The common occurrence of parental separation does not make this easy for a child: don't underestimate the potential impact. A review of research shows that, on average, 50% more children with separated parents have problems than children whose parents have not separated,[4] including:

➤ academic difficulties
➤ self-esteem
➤ popularity with other children
➤ behavioural difficulties
➤ anxiety
➤ depression.

Many children may recover over time from the initial distress and adjust to the new structure of the family: behavioural problems, for instance, dissipate to normal levels two years after parental separation (perhaps partly because half of these behaviour problems have been found to predate the separation by a matter of years). Some children may find their circumstances improved by the separation, for instance if domestic violence stops or the level of conflict in the home reduces. The majority of children, probably at least two-thirds, recover more or less completely, but a significant minority continue to be affected.

Another research review summarised over 200 studies of the impact of parental separation on children.[5] This found that children whose carers have separated have a higher probability than children in intact families of:
➤ living in poverty
➤ having inadequate or overcrowded accommodation
➤ performing less well in school
➤ having frequent accidents
➤ reporting physical health problems
➤ having symptoms of depression
➤ smoking cigarettes
➤ drinking alcohol to excess
➤ other substance misuse
➤ showing behavioural problems of concern to adults
➤ leaving school before school leaving age
➤ leaving home before the age of 18 years
➤ becoming sexually active before the age of 16 years
➤ becoming pregnant as a teenager
➤ becoming a parent as a teenager.

These cannot simply be attributed to the separation itself: other factors may have far more impact, including the nature of the situation before the separation and what happens afterwards.

Which children are least or most affected?
Factors contributing to a child's resilience in the face of parental separation include:
➤ the child's own temperament and resilience
➤ the child's ability to understand and make sense of what has happened, which partly depends on what sorts of explanation he has been given
➤ the remaining parent being resilient and resourceful – how others around the child adjust to the separation is of great importance to the child
➤ support from siblings
➤ support from extended family – grandparents in particular are a valued support
➤ support from friends of the remaining parent
➤ support from friends of the child
➤ support from school
➤ continuity of financial status
➤ not having to move house
➤ continuity at school

➤ how well the separated parents can get on with each other (without necessarily meeting each other)
➤ being able to maintain positive and regular contact with the absent parent.

This last factor may have particular salience for some children. Adolescents can find a lack of contact with the separated parent very difficult, so it is worrying that 28% of all children whose parents have separated have no contact with their fathers three years after the separation.[6] The exception seems to be that children of seriously violent or antisocial fathers do better without contact.

Factors that may make it more difficult for the child to adjust to his changed circumstances can be summarised as the following three main issues.

➤ *Financial difficulties* can be a major factor: being poorer is difficult for everyone. It is probably more difficult to cope with being poor if you have got used to being well off. The first thing that an abandoned parent needs may be financial, legal and housing advice, which may distract from focusing on the emotional needs of her children.
➤ The *relationship* between each child and each parent.
   – The parent with whom the child lives may find the new situation difficult to cope with, particularly if she has mental or physical health problems. Parental depression is more likely in unsupported single parents. Echoes of previous trauma may have a big impact, for instance in the case of the son who reminds his mother of his violent father (*see* Case Example in Box 9.1). The emotional impact of multiple losses or deaths may stack up. Any parent is likely to find the loss of an important relationship quite disorienting, and may experience bereavement-type symptoms such as disbelief, shock or anger – making it difficult to be emotionally available to support her child's emotional needs (*see* Case Example in Box 9.2).
   – The relationship with the absent parent is also important. Unpredictable changes in the level of contact, or promised contacts that don't materialise, can play havoc with the child's emotions.
➤ The child's experience of *conflict*:
   – between biological parents
   – between the child and a step-parent or parental cohabitee
   – between the remaining parent and any cohabitee.

BOX 9.1 Case Example

At the age of 11 years, Craig has begun to demonstrate increasingly aggressive behaviour towards his mother, Dora. His parents separated six months ago following domestic violence between them, mainly from his father, Luke, towards his mother. Craig finds the continuing rows between his parents distressing, though not as bad as when they were together. Dora takes him to the general practitioner, saying she wants him to have a brain scan because she thinks he must have the same thing wrong with his head as his father. Craig is an only child.

Dora tells their general practitioner that when Craig becomes aggressive, she can see Luke in him. His aggression reminds her so much of her ex-husband that it brings back past memories and she feels powerless in the same way that she did with Luke. The general practitioner helps her recognise that because of her fear that Craig will become like his father, and her guilt about what he has witnessed in the past, Dora is finding it difficult to set limits on Craig's behaviour, and tends to give in to his every demand. When she tries to say 'No', he responds just like a toddler would, to test what boundaries she can impose. He is not currently learning the consequences of his behaviour, particularly when he is aggressive. Although she feels this is all her fault, Dora knows her general practitioner well and trusts her, so is able to hear this – and it makes sense to her.

The general practitioner explains that Craig has half his genes in common with Luke, so his aggressive behaviour may be partly genetic, but it is very unlikely to show up on an ordinary brain scan. If they could get Craig and Luke into an ultra-modern scanner that showed what areas of the brain are most active when each of them is aggressive, and supposing these proved to be the same areas, this would not help much with managing the situation. The best way to improve Craig's behaviour would be to work out ways in which Dora can be firmer, and not let her guilt about what has happened make her give in to Craig's tantrums – while finding every opportunity to praise and reward Craig's good behaviour, and have some enjoyable shared activities.

The general practitioner suggests that Dora should attend a parenting group to help her learn in more detail how to achieve all this. She also suggests that Dora should have some support for herself from the practice counsellor, to focus perhaps on her coping strategies following the separation and her possible post-traumatic stress disorder. She also suggests that Dora should let Craig's head of year at his new secondary school know what has happened, as the staff there are not yet familiar with him.

Dora says she has found their conversation very helpful. She does not like groups very much and has a lot of support from her sister, who has four children. She will discuss the situation with the school, but rather than attending a parenting group or see the counsellor, she would like to try to put the general practitioner's advice into practice. They agree on a review appointment for three weeks, booked as double the usual length, since they have by now gone far in excess of time.

A developmental perspective: how children of different ages respond differently

A *preschool child* is even more likely to regress than the seven-year-old boy in the case example in Box 9.2.

➤ He may return to the parental bed after sleeping alone for some time.
➤ He may become more clingy or anxious about separating from carers.
➤ He may show confusion about the new situation, for instance by frequently searching for or asking about the absent parent.

BOX 9.2 Case Example

John is seven years old when his father, Antoine, leaves his mother, Gwen, for another woman. Gwen very much wants John's father back, and can't understand how this other woman has such a hold on him.

Gwen is visiting the practice nurse for a cervical swab when she mentions that John has recently been wetting the bed at night three to four times per week, having been dry since he was three years old. The practice nurse is fortunately already aware of the acrimonious separation, so asks Gwen about the impact on John. Gwen immediately starts talking about her own distress, and how betrayed she feels.

It emerges that Antoine has recently introduced John to his new partner. Gwen has asked John numerous questions about the relationship between Antoine and his other woman, most of which John cannot answer: all he is able to say is that: 'She seems all right'. The practice nurse also finds out that John's parents have been arguing recently over contact arrangements. She explains to Gwen that John seems to be getting caught up in grown-up stuff: if she cannot forgive Antoine or discuss practical things with him without their emotions erupting, then at least she needs to find a way of protecting John from all this.

They agree that the best way to deal with the bedwetting is to invest in a plastic mattress cover, remain calm and not make a fuss when the bedding has to be changed. Gwen asks whether there could be a physical cause; the practice nurse says this does not sound likely, but she gives Gwen a specimen pot for a urine sample to exclude an infection and says she will check with John's general practitioner whether any other tests are needed. They arrange a follow-up meeting in four weeks, but before Gwen leaves, she volunteers that Antoine has always got on well with her mother, so she thinks it might be better if she leaves the practical negotiations to her, and stops asking John questions about that 'other woman'. The practice nurse says that these sound like two very good ideas.

At the next meeting four weeks later, the practice nurse tells Gwen that the urine test shows no signs of infection. The general practitioner has said that no further tests are necessary in the circumstances, but if the bedwetting doesn't stop, John could be seen in the enuresis clinic, which includes a community paediatrician. However, it turns out that John's wetting has reduced to only once or twice per week. Gwen attributes this to the contact arrangements flowing more smoothly, and her making every effort to protect John from her feelings about Antoine.

Over the next two months, the bedwetting continues to reduce, then stops completely.

A ***child aged five to nine years*** is still not mature enough to understand the whole situation but is able to recognise that one parent has left and talk about this. He may be concerned that if one parent can go, so could the other. He is likely to want his parents to get back together – regardless of the prior situation. A child of this age is likely to experience the world as revolving around him (*egocentricity*), so may fashion an explanation of how the parental separation is due to something he has done (or not done): 'If I had not shouted at my dad the week before he left, he would have stayed'; or 'If I had done my homework like daddy told me to, he wouldn't have gone'.

An **older preadolescent** or **adolescent** is usually better able to understand the antecedents and consequences of a separation and think about how it could affect everyone's life. He is likely to struggle with feeling that the situation is out of his control – so will want to be involved in any decisions directly affecting him. Friendships outside the home become more important with increasing age, so leading to a greater impact from any change that disrupts friendships, such as geographical moves of home or school.

Reconstituted families

Parental separation may lead to family **reconstitution.** New members of the family may include:
➤ a parental cohabitee or step-parent
➤ the children of this new adult
➤ and (subsequently) new half-siblings.

Each of these changes to the family constitution could be seen as a further life-change requiring adjustment from each child. One child may see each such change as an exciting opportunity to start again, while another may find it an occasion for anxiety and/or rebellion. A **child's feelings** may include:
➤ resentment of decisions made without his input
➤ resentment at having to submit to the authority of a new adult
➤ pleasure at having new playmates
➤ disgruntlement at having to share (toys, rooms, time with particular adults ...)
➤ feeling displaced by the new children or step-children of the departed parent, feeling not as loved as before; or feeling disregarded
➤ disappointment at missed contacts or inadequate time with the absent parent
➤ a new-found sense of stability and security.

Each **parent**, particularly the new arrival, has to develop new relationships and set new household rules and boundaries: the balance of power may shift (*see also* Chapter 8 on Family Issues). The new cohabitee may be confused about how and when to parent his partner's children, how to show affection and even what to be called. There may be financial stresses, relating for instance to the need for larger accommodation or difficulties securing maintenance payments. On the positive side, the arrival of a new adult in the household may bring a new stability, for instance in terms of shared parenting, financial security and access to a wider family network of support.

Despite the potential difficulties and challenges, the reconstitution of families can bring many advantages for everyone, and usually settles in time.

ASSESSMENT

Who is seeking help? This will affect how you begin your assessment. Usually it is a parent worried by the effects of separation on one or more children; sometimes it is a teacher, noticing a change in the child's behaviour or achievement in school; or it may be a child approaching a professional directly.

Whoever makes the first contact, it is important to **understand** at least an outline of what has happened, and to focus on how this might seem from the point of view of each of the children, allowing for developmental stage. One way of clarifying the current family composition is to ask a child to help you draw a *family tree*. The following categories may help structure your questions.

➤ What happened **prior** to the separation? What did each child witness? Often children witness or are aware of far more than parents realise – and may feel responsible for not stopping it. The prior parental relationship can range from domestic violence to no apparent conflict: the separation may be a complete surprise to one parent. Other life events may affect everyone's adjustment to the separation, such as parental illness, a death in the family or financial stresses.

➤ How did the **separation itself** happen? In particular, how was each child informed? How much has he been told? Was the explanation age-appropriate? What was each child led to expect would happen as a result of the separation?

➤ What is happening as a **consequence** of the separation? What sort of losses has each child had to endure, such as friendships, relatives or pets? What contact arrangements have been agreed with the departed parent and close relatives on his side of the family, such as paternal grandparents or others who have been important for the child? How easy has it been to agree the amount and nature of contact? Are there good reasons for limiting or preventing contact? Have the parents been able to communicate calmly about such issues?

➤ Has there been **professional involvement**, such as solicitors, the court, mediation, Relate or the Child and Family Court Advisory and Support Service (CAFCASS)? If so, has this improved the situation for each child (as any form of mediation should do) or has it increased the antagonism between parents (as the adversarial process that characterises legal proceedings is liable to do). Be wary of any attempts to involve you in the legal process: it is best to keep separate the roles of professional helper and professional assessor.

➤ **How is each child adjusting** to his changed circumstances? If this does not become apparent from the conversation, you can probe about the child's involvement in and ability to enjoy activities such as homework, time with friends and spare-time interests.

➤ **How is each parent adjusting** to the separation? Is either of them finding it difficult to cope? How well are they communicating together? Are they exposing any of the children to continuing conflict? Are they using any of the children as a spy or go-between (meaning the main channel of communication between parents who won't speak to each other directly)? Are any of the children being enrolled as an ally in an ongoing battle? Are any of the children becoming young carers for one of the adults?

BOX 9.3 Alarm Bells in assessment following parental separation

Significant losses for the child in addition to the separation
Past or continuing domestic violence
Ongoing conflict between parents
Parental distress or difficulty coping
Parental isolation and lack of support
Child isolation and lack of support
Evident deterioration in child's functioning at home or at school

MANAGEMENT AND REFERRAL

A large variety of professionals may be asked for – and should be able to give – advice about how to cope following parental separation. This should not usually require referral for specialist input. As well as giving some of the following suggested advice, you can direct parents to the leaflets, books and websites listed in the Resources section below.

A parent may be worried that separation or divorce may permanently damage her children, perhaps because she feels this happened to her as a child. In this situation, false reassurances that everything will be all right may be unhelpful, but you could say that life after separation can be just as good as before, or even better, if both parents work hard to make it so. Points to emphasise include the following.

➤ Ongoing **conflict** between parents, particularly if it is witnessed by a child, is likely to have a detrimental effect – both through its direct emotional impact, and indirectly, by undermining contact arrangements. Parents need to find a way of *not* arguing, even if this means severely limiting any communication between them, as in the case example in Box 9.2. The children's needs and interests will be best served by both parents being able to communicate and agree about the priorities for each child – which usually means putting antagonism to one side.

➤ **Contact** should be regular and predictable. How often contacts should occur and for how long depend on what is practically possible, including geographical factors, as well as the ages and wishes of each child. A younger child may find it easier to manage shorter, more frequent contacts, whereas an adolescent may prefer longer-lasting contacts, such as a week or two during school holidays, but less frequently. A common pattern is for children to visit the absent parent for part of every other weekend, but this is not necessarily suitable for everyone. Some parents are both able to remain close enough to each child's school to share the week fairly equally. It is remarkable how well most children will tolerate *any* arrangement as long as it is clearly agreed by the relevant adults and becomes reliable. It may however be worth warning parents that most children show more challenging behaviour (or some degree of emotional upset) after returning from contact with the absent parent (and sometimes just before

going): this does *not* meant that the contact is a *bad thing*. It can be explained in terms of the child having to make all sorts of adjustments, such as to:
— the different sets of rules in each household
— the need to test boundaries
— the new members of each household
— the journey each way
— possessions left in the other house
— friends not close enough to the other house
— his divided loyalties to each parent
— a need to test how much each parent still loves him.
➤ Each child needs to preserve his relationship with each parent as far as possible. In situations of domestic violence or child abuse this may not be possible, but otherwise, each parent should make as much effort as possible to **say only positive things** about the other parent, and avoid expressing the criticism they are likely to feel in front of the children. Openly expressed derogatory comments can lead to confused feelings for the child, who may have conflicting loyalties or feel torn between the two parental viewpoints. Ideally, each child should be encouraged to love each parent – which will make it easier for him in turn to feel loved.

BOX 9.4 Case Example

Following their separation, Jeremy and Cynthia are both determined to do their best for their children, Natalia (aged nine years) and Alfie (aged six years), and to share the parenting duties as equally as possible. So the children stay with Jeremy for alternate weekends and Tuesday and Thursday nights, and with Cynthia on alternate weekends and Monday and Wednesday nights. Although there are some difficulties agreeing upon this routine and getting the children to accept it, after about six months everything appears to run smoothly. The children seem to be happy at school and accept that they have two different homes.

BOX 9.5 Case Example

Kaho, aged seven years, lives with his mother and three elder half-sisters. His father, Dexter, has been living so far away that they have had no direct contact for two years, but now Dexter has returned to live three streets away. Kaho expects that Dexter will now be able to see him regularly. Dexter bumps into Kaho in the street and promises to come round for his birthday the following week. Unfortunately, Dexter's new partner resents his having any contact with Kaho or his mother, so the promised contact seldom materialises. Kaho becomes repeatedly disappointed by such broken promises, and his behaviour noticeably deteriorates.

➤ Although much change is inevitable, parents should *keep as many things the same as possible*, to help the child feel that his world is safe and predictable, and that his life can continue as before. For example, the child should carry on with normal routines (such as at bedtime and on school-day mornings) and with activities he enjoys (such as after-school clubs, weekend sport, or visits to grandparents or cousins). Maintaining several small but salient parts of a child's life can be an example of little things making a big difference.

BOX 9.6 Case Example

Felicity is concerned that her three children are much more difficult to manage when they return from their father's. She therefore stops them seeing him. He applies to the court, which directs the Child and Family Court Advisory and Support Service (CAFCASS) to assess the advisability of the children having contact with him. Professionals from this organisation carry out an assessment. This includes meeting with each child alone and setting up an observed contact between all three of them and their father at the local contact centre. Their conclusion is that the father has a good relationship with all three children, and can cope with them well when they see him together, so contact should continue. After this is debated in court, the judge directs that the children should visit their father for staying contact every other weekend, and should spend at least one third of the school holidays and half-terms with him.

➤ Children need to be *kept informed* about what is happening. It is not always easy to decide how much to tell each child, but each explanation needs to be age-appropriate, and each child needs to know enough to make sense of what is happening – without feeling it is his fault. A younger child in particular needs reassurance that he is not going to be abandoned by the remaining parent and that the separation is not his fault. An adolescent may need a fuller explanation that involves sharing painful truths, such as the involvement of overlapping relationships in leading to the separation. It may be best to build on the adaptation that will occur over time by gradually revealing more of the whole picture. Questions should be answered as honestly as possible at any age, even if the answer is: 'You will have to ask your father that'.
➤ *Others* may also *need to be kept informed*, including for instance key teachers at school, leaders of clubs outside school and any relatives who have contact with the child. These adults need to know how to interpret any changes in behaviour or emotional expression.
➤ Parents need to accept the need for each child to *show* his *emotions* in his own way, providing this does not damage anyone.
➤ Children need to be *consulted* about changes. This does not mean giving a five-year-old child the power to decide which parent he lives with (to take an extreme example); it may, however, be appropriate to ask older adolescents to make this sort of decision. In general, each child should be given an opportunity to

express his views about an important change while making it clear that the decision will be made by the adults (which, if parents cannot agree, may sometimes mean the judge!). Sometimes the situation is so fraught for parents that a child may find it easier to talk to another adult, such as a less emotionally involved relative, a close friend (adult or adolescent), a trusted professional (perhaps at school), or a dedicated agency such as Relateen (the usual title for the children's branch of Relate), which unfortunately is available only in some areas.[7]

➤ Parents *should be advised not to*:
  — use any child as a message carrier
  — use any child as a spy
  — allow any child to become a pawn in a battle with the ex-partner.

➤ In some situations *a child can begin to take on the role of the absent partner* – either by becoming the main companion for a lonely parent or actually looking after a parent who is sick, depressed or using too much alcohol or other substances. A mother may say to her son: 'You are the only man in the house now'; or keep the eldest child up late to have some company in the evening. This situation is not always easy to handle, particularly as the child may be very concerned, having lost one parent, about losing the other – so may be clingy or over-attentive to the remaining parent. Sometimes gentle conversation with the remaining parent may help clarify the respective roles of adult and child, emphasising the child's developmental stage. The parent may need some nudging to find alternative sources of support from friends or professionals or local support groups such as Gingerbread.[8] An adolescent may be able to take on some of the household chores, but needs also to be able to focus on school and the development of his own friendships. A younger child needs to be clear that his parent is not his responsibility – which will be possible only if she takes on responsibility for herself.

➤ Some parents may feel guilty about the separation (whether justifiably or not) and may therefore **overcompensate** by buying lots of gifts, taking the child out on lots of activities, or relaxing rules. Although the extra time and attention may be valuable to the child, substituting material things for this is not, and increased laxity may be harmful. What each child needs is a continuing sense of containment and stability: maintaining the same limits to behaviour can help sustain this, as can regular and predictable quality time – which does not need to involve going out or spending money.

Although you cannot predict that everything will be all right in a certain number of months or years, most children's **adjustment** to parental separation **does settle over time**. Helping parents see the normality of the situation – or at least how common such adjustment difficulties are – may help them sidestep any guilty feelings and take on board the advice that is available from many sources.

Although the majority of parents should benefit from such advice, some families may need **referral** to specialist services, for instance if one of the children has become significantly depressed, or if the child's behavioural difficulties need further assessment.

BOX 9.7 Practice Points for management following parental separation

Encourage parents to find a way of communicating about each child if possible

Focus on each child's point of view

The child's behaviour or emotions may be entirely understandable in the circumstances

If a parent's needs make it difficult to prioritise the needs of the children, then try to find a way of meeting the parent's needs

RESOURCES
Leaflets
- The Royal College of Psychiatrists factsheets on mental health and growing up: *Divorce or separation of parents – the impact on children and adolescents: information for parents, carers and anyone who works with young people.* Available at: www.rcpsych.ac.uk/mentalhealthinfo/mentalhealthandgrowingup/divorceandseparation.aspx (accessed 24 March 2011).
- Young Minds downloadable publications: *Keeping in touch – guide on separation and divorce for parents.* Available at: www.youngminds.org.uk/publications/all-publications/keeping-in-touch (accessed 24 March 2011).

Websites
- Action for Children has set up: www.itsnotyourfault.org
- Divorce Aid: www.divorceaid.co.uk
- Families Need Fathers: www.fnf.org.uk

Organisations
- Relate is a voluntary organisation that can mediate before or after parental separation: www.relate.org.uk. Some branches have a component called Relateen that offers help specifically to young people affected by parental separation.
- National Family Mediation: www.nfm.org.uk
- The National Stepfamily Association has been taken over by Parentline Plus, which in turn has been subsumed into Family Lives: http://familylives.org.uk/advice/stepfamilies

Books for children
- Cole J. *My Parents' Divorce (Thoughts and Feelings)*. London: Franklin Watts; 2007.
  This book for children of four to eight years discusses why divorce happens and how to cope with the difficult feelings that arise.
- Fine A. *Step by Wicked Step*. London: Puffin; 2001.
  Five children gather around a mysterious diary and share an evening of stories about their lives and trials, discovering common bonds in adversity. This is a story about the effects of divorce and remarriage upon children.
- Lavette S. *Step Families (Talking About)*. London: Franklin Watts; 2007.
- Stones R. *Children Don't Divorce (Talking it Through)*. London: Happy Cat Books; 2002.
  This can be a good book to read to a child to help her through the break-up of her family: it is a well-illustrated picture book, and may help a young child to know that he or she is not the only child in the world who has parents who have stopped loving each other.

- Wilson J, Sharrat N. *Suitcase Kid*. London: Corgi Yearling Book; 2006.
  A story for children of nine to 12 years about a girl and her tiny stuffed rabbit adjusting to the difficulties of having divorced parents and her life of joint custody.

Books for parents

- Burrett J. *To and Fro Children: a guide to successful parenting after divorce*. 3rd ed. London: Carrington Psychology; 1999.
- De'Ath E, Slater D, Fell S, *et al. Parenting Threads: Caring for Children When Couples Part*. London: National Stepfamily Association; 1992.
  This provides practical advice for families wanting to prioritise the children after parental separation.

REFERENCES

1 Rodgers B, Pryor J. *Divorce and Separation: the outcomes for children*. York: Joseph Rowntree Foundation; 1998.
2 Office of National Statistics. *Divorces in England and Wales 2008*. London: Office of National Statistics; 2008. Available at: www.statistics.gov.uk/pdfdir/div0110.pdf (accessed 24 March 2011).
3 Layard R, Dunn J. *A Good Childhood: searching for values in a competitive age*. London: The Children's Society and Penguin Books; 2009. pp. 13–32.
4 Ibid.
5 Rodgers, op. cit.
6 Layard, op. cit.
7 www.relate.org.uk/young-people-counselling/index.html
8 www.gingerbread.org.uk

CHAPTER 10

Death, dying and bereavement

INTRODUCTION

Before the age of 18 years, most individuals will experience the emotional impact of at least one death: this may be of a close family member, relative, friend, friend's relative or pet. Most children and young people will manage the grieving process satisfactorily, with support from those around them. However, for others the process can be more difficult and at times devastating. Referrals to child and adolescent mental health services are often made or considered when the child appears to be struggling to come to terms with the loss or is not acting in a manner that the surrounding adults feel comfortable with. Often, therapeutic input is not required and it is sufficient to confirm that the child's behaviour is part of a normal grieving process; parents may benefit from support, information or advice. Sometimes, a child's adjustment to the loss or the family's ability to support the child can be impaired, in which case additional help may be required. This could include, for instance: discussion with the family to enhance the surviving adults' understanding of the child's feelings, direct support or therapeutic input for the child or other family members, or referral to a specialist service.

A child's adjustment to a loved one's terminal illness, her own mortality or a death is in part dependent upon her understanding of the concept of death. This is influenced by her previous experience of death, her developmental level and the amount and type of support around the child. When thinking about what, if anything, to do, it is important to find out what the child, her family and others around her have said about the death and to attempt an understanding of the family's religious and cultural attitudes to death. In our society, death can often be a taboo subject that adults may be reluctant to talk about, especially to children.

A developmental perspective: the child's concept of death

A child's understanding of death gradually increases with age. Piaget's Theory of cognitive development[1] can help to explain how a child requires certain cognitive skills to understand fully the finality and universality of death (*see* Box 10.1). This is true in general, but different children develop emotionally at different rates, and some children may develop their concepts of death in response to individual experiences, particularly if these are mediated helpfully by the surrounding family.

BOX 10.1 Piaget's model of how children think applied to the maturation of ideas about death and dying

> **Preoperational Stage – birth to seven years:** Children's thinking about events is based upon what they see rather than logical or rational thought processes. Most do not understand that death is permanent and final. At this stage, the child tends to be egocentric, seeing herself as the cause of, or reason, for everything that happens – which increases the risk of 'magical thinking' – for instance attributing a death or departure to something the child did or thought.
>
> **Concrete Operational Stage – seven to 11 years:** Children now understand that causes and consequences are regularly linked, and have increased understanding of the irreversibility and universality of death. They continue to struggle with abstract ideas or hypothetical propositions that do not seem clearly based in reality.
>
> **Formal Operational Stage – 11 to 16 years:** Young people are developing abstract and hypothetical thought, and can therefore appreciate general rules, such as that everyone will die.

Preoperational stage: birth to seven years; the child does not understand that death is permanent and final

One of the key areas during this stage of development is a child's ability to understand the irreversibility of death, namely that death is permanent and final. Very young children will <u>not</u> have developed this understanding and may present with a variety of behaviours that are often confusing for the adults around the child. A very young child can have awareness that the deceased person is missing and may show searching behaviour and distress. A child between the ages of three to seven years may be able to say quite clearly, 'My mummy is dead' but later may say, 'I hope she is back in time for my birthday party'.

Some children in this age range may confuse death with sleep and consequently may worry about dying when they go to sleep, or what will happen to the dead person when they wake up. This can be further complicated if children in this age group are given explanations about the death such as: 'They are going to sleep forever', or 'They are going on a long journey'. This can lead young children to develop fears of falling asleep or separation anxiety from caregivers out of the fear that they too may go on a long journey and not return. Given this, *children in this age group generally benefit from being given simple explanations about illness and death in words that they understand*. It also helps if they are given the same, not different, explanations by all around them.

Another key feature of a child's thinking during this developmental phase is *'magical thinking'*. The child thinks that her own thoughts, wishes or actions can cause things to happen; that something she thought or did caused the death; or that if she thinks or does something then the loved-one may return. The child may blame herself for a death if she had been feeling angry towards the loved one or may believe: 'If I am really, really good then mummy will come back'. *It is essential to tell the child that nothing they thought, said or did caused the death to occur.* They may need to be told, at regular intervals, that the death was not their fault. It may also be necessary to emphasise that the loved one will not return, whatever anyone does.

Concrete operational stage: seven to 11 years; the child has an increased understanding of the irreversibility and universality of death

During this developmental stage children tend to have a greater understanding of the irreversibility of death and are beginning to develop an understanding of the universality of death. Despite this they may still struggle to comprehend that death could actually happen to them, or to people who are not ill or old.

It is common in this age group for children to need details and appropriate facts about a terminal illness or death. They may ask lots of questions about how and why a person died and what will happen exactly to the person's dead body. Questions about how a body decomposes are not uncommon, or when a cremation is to occur how this takes place. A child in this age group may learn about death from a variety of sources such as: home, school, adults or children within the same religion or not, friends or neighbours. It is important to find out what the child already knows and believes, in order to add to it rather than risk contradicting powerful beliefs. In response to a child's questions, it is important to try to be as honest as possible – providing you have parental permission, for instance for divulging that a loved one has an illness that may well lead to death. It is also important to frame any answers in appropriately simple language, with vocabulary and amount of information tailored to the child's level of understanding. *Parents may need help to understand that the child's questions may be different from theirs and that it is alright to talk to a child about illness and death.*

During this developmental stage, a child is also becoming increasingly aware of other people's emotional states and coping skills. She may hold onto her own confusion and questions out of a fear that these might further upset the adults around her. The child may construe a lack of adult conversation about the death as a sign that the adults cannot cope with such conversations – leading the child to hold onto her own thoughts, some of which may be unhelpful. In addition, she may construe the appropriate adult expression of normal grieving emotions, such as anger or sadness, as a sign of weakness. It is therefore helpful for children in this age range to be reassured that there is no right or wrong way to grieve and that the strength of their emotions is normal, and to be given explicit permission to talk, ask questions and demonstrate a range of feelings.

Formal operational stage: 11 to 16 years; the child understands that everyone will die

This is the stage in which a child fully begins to appreciate the universality of death. The emotional significance of the inevitability of one's own death develops over a lifetime.

During adolescence, peers tend to assume greater importance, and there is a natural separation from family. Some carers may interpret this behaviour as an avoidance strategy, or an inability to access the support available from within the family – in which case, it may be helpful for the professional to point out how normal it is for the adolescent to seek support from friends rather than exclusively from family.

In addition, normal adolescence entails an increase in risk-taking behaviours, sometimes in response to peer or media pressure, such as: experimenting with drugs or alcohol, exploring murky corners of the Internet, or engaging in minor criminality or self-harming behaviours. After bereavement, it can be hard to know whether an increase in risk-taking behaviour is part of the grieving process or would have happened anyway. Whatever the true explanation, it may be helpful to address these behaviours (rather than dismiss them as just a phase) and to discuss with the adolescent alternative strategies for expressing himself or coping with feelings.

During adolescence, physical and hormonal changes occur that can have a significant impact upon mood. It is therefore common for adolescents to find the strength and intensity of their emotions both confusing and frightening. The expectations of adults around the adolescent may also be important, for instance about how emotions are managed, or what responsibilities are age-appropriate. Following a death, some adolescents are expected to manage their emotions like an adult and may even be given adult responsibilities. This may be very frightening or bewildering even for an apparently mature adolescent.

Alongside the turbulence arising from a variety of emotions may be some cognitive reactions – given the adolescent's increasing understanding and ability to consider abstract and hypothetical reasoning. These may include, for instance: an understanding of others' reactions to the loss, a prediction of the consequences of the loss for self and others, or an attribution of responsibility for the death: 'I should have stopped my mum from drinking', or 'I should have told someone that my mum was depressed', or 'It was because I had a row with dad that he went out and got run over by a speeding car'. Such self-blame is likely to be very unhelpful, and should be addressed by the surviving adults, with help if necessary from any involved professional – with an understanding that the self-blaming cognitions may be difficult to shift.

MODELS OF LOSS: THE GRIEF PROCESS IN CHILDREN AND ADOLESCENTS
It used to be thought that children did not grieve or that their grief was very different from an adult's. However, we now know that children do grieve and experience similar feelings to adults. There are several theoretical models that can help us to understand the process of grief and loss.

The most well known of these models is the **Stage Model of Loss**,[2] which suggests that an individual passes through various stages following a bereavement before successfully resolving most of the feelings about the death. These *stages* include:
➤ shock
➤ denial

➤ anger
➤ guilt
➤ depression
➤ resolution.

Individuals do not pass through these stages in a fixed order and can go back and forth through different stages repeatedly. Grief resists being regimented.

The **Task Model of Loss**[3] is similar in that it suggests children (specifically) go through *four psychological tasks* to reach a resolution:
➤ understanding
➤ grieving
➤ commemorating
➤ moving on.

A further model called the **Dual Process Model** describes grief as a *dynamic process* with individuals oscillating between focusing on the *loss* and *avoidance* of the loss experience.[4]

Having an understanding of the above models can help us to recognise the range of emotions children and their families can experience. In reality, families often describe an even wider range of emotions than is recognised in the models, including: sadness, anger, frustration, guilt, loneliness, despair, shame, powerlessness, disbelief, feeling frozen, numbness, worthlessness, and (hardly surprisingly amidst the maelstrom of all these feelings) confusion. In addition, these emotions may not always be related to the experience of death itself but to a variety of consequences of the death. For example, it is common after the death of one parent for the surviving parent to feel inadequate: 'I can't even keep up with the bills; he was always the one that dealt with the money'. Children may experience a deterioration in financial circumstances or an undesired house move.

Helping children and families to understand the normality of what they are going through can often make it easier for them to cope with the array of feelings and may enable parents to understand the consequent changes in their children's behaviour. The dual process model can be very helpful in recognising how normal it is to dip in and out of grief. Some individuals may react to entirely normal periods of enjoyment after losing a loved one with overwhelming feelings of guilt. Some may feel they ought to be spending more time thinking about the deceased. This oscillation between periods of disregard for the death and periods of grieving for the loss may be particularly apparent in children and can be reflected in their behaviour. For example, a child may switch rapidly from being extremely distressed and sad about the loss of a loved one while talking to a teacher to running around the school playground with her peers with every appearance of enjoyment.

Factors affecting the grief process

Many factors may affect the grieving process for the child and family.

Cultural expectations, religious beliefs and cultural traditions affect how a child or family manage a terminal illness and how the survivors grieve for the loss of a loved one. For example, some cultures have a specified mourning period and are expected to dress and act in a certain manner during this time period. Within the family's own culture, there may be family beliefs about the proper length of mourning and how this should be done. Some traditions and rituals may be very helpful in facilitating families' grief; others may be less so, for instance the belief by some parents that children should never be taken to funerals (thus depriving them of an opportunity for some group-supported ritual mourning).

Factors that can affect the quality and intensity of the grieving process include the following:

➤ *the nature of the death*: For example, was it gradual and expected or sudden and unexpected? Was it the result of natural causes, suicide or homicide?
➤ *multiple losses*: A death in the family may be particularly hard to bear if any other close family members have died within the last few years.
➤ *consequential losses* may affect family members adversely, such as a reduction in family income, complex legal issues, the loss of the family home or a change in school. (Not all consequences are negative: one or more deaths may lead to an increase in closeness between surviving family members; life insurance payouts may improve the family's financial situation.)
➤ *child temperament and resilience* (*see* Chapters 5 and 6). A child may be predisposed to deal well or poorly with disappointing life events.[5]
➤ *parental personality and resilience*: The child will find the adjustment easier if the remaining carer or carers also adjust well.
➤ *attachment*: The child with a secure attachment to remaining caregivers may cope better with the loss of one of her attachment figures.
➤ *relationship with dead person*: The type of relationship the child had with the lost loved-one.
➤ *social factors*: Does the family's social network provide adequate support for the child and surviving carer(s)? Are there mental or physical health issues affecting those around the child, substance misuse or domestic violence?

Loss of a sibling

The loss of a sibling is likely to cause sadness and loneliness in surviving children, but parents should be aware that there may well be mixed feelings. A surviving sibling may feel a sense of pleasure at now having more exclusive attention from parents. It is also common for a child to feel guilty that something she has said, thought or done may have caused the death of her sibling.

The parent's reaction to the loss will have a significant impact on how the remaining children cope. If the parent is preoccupied with the dead child, the survivors may be deprived of love and attention. Parents may consciously or unconsciously blame them for being alive. Other parental reactions include becoming overprotective of a surviving child, or idealising the child who has died and so setting impossible standards for those who remain.

Bereavement by suicide

Bereavement following suicide is traumatic, and the feelings of guilt, shame, stigma, rejection and isolation set it apart from the sadness following other forms of death and can make it harder for surviving relatives to seek help. They are more likely to need professional support of some sort, are at increased risk of abnormal grief reactions, and may be more at risk of suicide themselves. It is suggested that for each completed suicide, an average of six surrounding individuals are deeply affected, including children. The *Help is at Hand* booklet has been developed for people bereaved by suicide, those who support them and professionals dealing with bereaved individuals.[6]

ASSESSMENT

When carrying out an assessment to assist in deciding what professional input, if any, may help or support a bereaved family, it is important to consider as many of the aforementioned factors as you can. Once you have established a broader picture, it should be easier to agree with the family whether any intervention is required, and if so what.

Who is concerned and why? Who is asking for help or advice? Is it staff at the child's school? If so, what are their main concerns? Is it the health visitor or general practitioner? If so, who has asked them to seek further help? Is it the surviving carer? Are the main concerns about behavioural or emotional expression – or lack of emotional expression? Is it possible to work out from these concerns whether the picture is likely to be part of normal grief or something outside this?

Find out about the death. Who died? How and when? How did the child or children (and family) find out? What has the child been told? What questions have the children been asking?

Find out how the child who is giving rise to concern has been getting on recently at school. Has there been any deterioration in her learning or change in behaviour, and over what period? For many children, school can be an escape from the reality of a terminal illness or the loss of a loved one, so they may wish to preserve at school a pretence that everything is the same as before the illness or death. But since children spend a considerable amount of their waking hours at school, teachers or other school staff are likely to have observed some changes, and may have questions or concerns of their own.

Find out what support networks exist around the family, and whether there are any other agencies already involved. Possibilities include the local hospice, the paediatric palliative care team, social services and the health visitor. How do any involved professionals see the family as coping? What is the communication style of the family? Resilient families with close confiding relationships, effective social supports and good relationships with their extended family are likely to cope better with any bereavement.

If you can get most of this information, then even without meeting the child or family, you may be able to decide whether they appear to be grieving appropriately with the information and support they need, or whether further advice or help is warranted.

BOX 10.2 Alarm Bells in the assessment suggesting an excessive grief reaction or at least that help or referral is indicated

A persistent deterioration in academic performance and social functioning
Continued denial/disbelief regarding the death beyond the first few months
Suicidal ideation or feelings of hopelessness
Ongoing separation anxiety or school refusal
Mental health difficulties in carers
Development of fears and phobias that impair functioning
Recurrent or persisting somatic symptoms
Taboos in the family about discussing the death, and avoidance of culturally appropriate rituals

MANAGEMENT

General principles

The *primary goal* in the grieving process is the *acceptance of the reality and irreversibility of the death*. Only once this task has been achieved can the child or family process the emotional impact of the death and begin to reach a resolution.

It is important to give children and families the message that it is vital to have the space to talk about the terminal illness or death and the resulting losses. *Giving a child permission to talk* may be crucial – particularly after the initial few months, when others around the child may not directly ask about the loss of her loved one. A child may feel isolated when she is not able to talk, or have fantasises that others around her have forgotten her loved one or the impact of the experience on her.

The impact of a terminal illness or death in a family should never be underestimated. In some instances, the surviving adults in the family may be struggling to come to terms with their own grief or losses experienced as a consequence of the death (such as housing issues or financial difficulties): if so, this may affect their parenting capacity. If the child's needs are not being met, then referral on to other agencies may become essential, even if parents are reluctant: for all workers in child mental health, the welfare of the child is paramount.[7]

The timing of input can vary greatly. In supporting families coming to terms with a terminal illness and managing the future loss it can be helpful to offer support early. This does not necessarily mean intensive or long-term work, as the level of input should be adjusted to the particular family's needs and wishes. Early input, if available and carefully tailored, can facilitate the involvement of children in the process and support carers in achieving this. This in turn may obviate future crisis interventions or complicated grief reactions.

UNDERSTANDING

Use the assessment framework above to gain an understanding of a family's needs and communication styles, and work out whether any professional input is required: in many cases, the child and family may be best left to their own reserves of coping, supported by their extended family, social network and cultural or religious beliefs.

EXPLANATION

What children need (*see* above) is information and age-appropriate explanations about what happened and what is going to happen in the future.

Understanding the cause of death can help a child cope with loss. Simple explanations about part of the body being too poorly for the doctors to fix, or discussions about ageing or accidents, can be adapted to the age of the child. There is a risk that if the cause of death is not clearly explained, children may feel the death is their responsibility. Before death, for instance with a chronic illness, children may also need adequate explanations, and the opportunity to visit the parent/sibling in hospital, even if this is not openly stated as a chance to say goodbye.

After the death, it may be more difficult for surrounding adults to attend to the needs of the child, and age-appropriate explanations of all the bewildering things that are happening may be forgotten or actively avoided. Simple changes in the child's life may become very important: 'Who is going to take me to school now that mummy is dead?' Sometimes all that is required is to facilitate a discussion about these issues between the child and her carers.

Explanations may involve religious ideas, but these need to be consistent with family beliefs. It may be confusing for a child to be fobbed off with a phrase such as: 'Mummy has gone to Heaven' in a family where this is not part of their religious belief, and the child may not even have heard the word 'Heaven' before. Young children view God and Heaven in very concrete ways, and introducing abstract religious concepts may cause problems if the family has had no prior belief or discussion about these ideas.

MOURNING

Children should be given the option of sharing in the family's mourning process where possible. Group rituals and ceremony can be very important for everyone. Children should be encouraged to talk about the dead loved one if they want to, and should be provided with mementoes such as photographs or special objects. It may also be helpful for everyone in the family to develop some way of marking (and thereby emotionally processing) each anniversary, especially for the first few years. This may be as simple as a family visit to the grave, plaque or place where the ashes have been scattered. Avoiding anniversaries, so as not to upset the child, may only lead the child to feel others have forgotten the loved one or they do not have permission for some reason to speak about the loss. Children should be encouraged to think about how they would like to remember the loved one and what they would like to do on the anniversary.

SECURITY

Following the loss of a parent, the mental health and ability to cope of the surviving parent has a major impact on the emotional well-being of the children. If the main caregiver dies, then the child may need to build a relationship with a new carer, and it is important that this develops into a stable solid relationship (if it is not already) to allow the child to feel secure. Children may attempt to look after the surviving parent, but while love and help should be accepted, the parent must make it clear who is caring and who is cared for. They may need help to re-establish their own support network too.

Professional input may include:

➤ *signposting* surviving carers to information, support networks, useful reading or appropriate websites
➤ *direct support* to the family and/or child. The amount and duration of this is variable, and different families may have different needs
➤ giving reassurance that the child is grieving appropriately and that family members are supporting the child effectively
➤ a neutral outsider to listen to their experience
➤ a discussion with carers about how to facilitate the child's grieving process
➤ individual work with the child
➤ discussions including the whole family (family work or family therapy)
➤ *referral* to another agency.

There is no right or wrong way to grieve, and no right or wrong way of supporting families. Each family will have different needs.

Direct work with children and families

When working directly with children and families the key goals should be:

➤ to listen actively
➤ to facilitate communication between family members
➤ to contain the resulting emotions (meaning that it feels safe to express quite difficult emotions, and that they can be discussed without fear of being overwhelmed by them).

Some families find talking difficult, for a variety of reasons, so direct work, particularly with younger children, may require the use of non-verbal forms of expression. Box 10.3 lists some creative ways of helping families through this difficult period.

BOX 10.3 Activities to support the grieving process

A variety of verbal and non-verbal techniques can be used either during a terminal illness or after a death. Examples include the following.

● Help the terminally ill parent write letters for special future life events (for instance, a child's 18th birthday, or the birth of their own children).
● Find age-appropriate ways of explaining to the child about the illness and how death occurs, what looking at a dead body may involve, and what happens at a funeral.

- Create a memory box – containing photos, mementoes, pieces of clothing, jewellery or other items important to the child or family.
- Develop a family record: this may include a family tree, funny stories about together times and records of happy memories, all potentially linked to photographs.
- Develop farewell rituals such as sending messages on helium balloons, planting a tree or scattering the ashes in a special place. Ask surviving children to devise a ceremony.
- Write messages for the deceased loved-one; for instance: 'If I could spend five minutes with mum this is what I would say:…'
- Work through a workbook on bereavement with the family or child.
- Use drawing or puppets with a child to explore what the death means.

With younger children, it is important to fashion jointly a story – pitched at the child's developmental level – about the terminal illness or death. This should enable any magical thinking (such as 'Mummy got ill because I wouldn't put my toys away') to be gently corrected. With slightly older children, it may be more appropriate to provide plenty of space and opportunity in the joint activity or conversation for the child to take the lead in generating questions. These should then be answered (perhaps by the professional or perhaps by a carer) as honestly as they deem suitable. For this age group and upwards, concrete evidence of the death will be a significant help to the grieving process. This can include for instance:

➤ being kept informed about the progress of a terminal illness
➤ looking at the dead body
➤ attending the funeral
➤ helping to scatter the ashes
➤ visiting the grave or plaque.

The child should be as involved as much as possible in the decision-making process about what is best for her to attend or not to attend. This can help her feel that she has at least some control, particularly over the speed at which she faces the reality of the death.

Direct work with families involves first selecting who should be involved in meetings. This may initially include only the child and one surviving carer, or everyone remaining in the household, or several people important to the child who have been affected by the death: this may mean, for instance, including a grandparent who does not live in the family home but has frequent contact or a caregiving role. Deciding whom to invite should if possible be a joint decision between the professional, the child and the carer(s). Pacing the discussion is important: although it may be possible to have a complete factual discussion of the nature and circumstances of the death in one session, this may unleash feelings that are too overwhelming. It may therefore be prudent to begin the discussion with the present situation, and focus initially on present feelings and relationships, so that the conversation remains tolerable, and is experienced as a relief and a release rather than a blow in the solar plexus. Remember that it is probably better to leave the family members to rely on their own resources to discuss things at home unless things have got so problematic that some facilitation of communication is required.

If the grieving process is giving the child some difficulties, then communication with the network of professionals around the family may be needed. Liaison with school may be particularly important (with consent from the child and carer). School staff can provide a great deal of stability and support for a child, but may need to be kept informed and given hints on how they can help. Keeping schools updated on key events such as anniversaries can enable them to be proactive or at least to make allowances for any associated behavioural changes. Class teachers or pastoral support teachers may be grateful to discuss how best to manage distress in the classroom, impaired academic achievement, difficult questions from peers or bullying.

REFERRAL

Counselling or other therapeutic input is not usually necessary for bereaved children, providing the surviving family members or other carers are themselves sufficiently resilient to help each child. If a child has major behavioural problems or symptoms of depression, then referral may be necessary, for instance to:

➤ a palliative care team
➤ a voluntary agency such as Winston's Wish
➤ a bereavement counsellor with experience of dealing with children – sometimes accessible through CRUSE
➤ a Tier 3 child and adolescent mental health service.

BOX 10.4 Case Example

A health visitor asks to discuss Stephanie, aged six years, with the primary child and adolescent mental health worker. Stephanie's father died very suddenly of a heart attack four months ago – which was a great shock for the whole family. The health visitor is already involved with the family because of Stephanie's one-year-old sister, and has agreed with the rest of the primary care team to remain the main support for the family. Concern about Stephanie has increased recently because of poor attendance at school, which has led to the educational welfare officer visiting.

The health visitor tells the primary child and adolescent mental health worker that Stephanie has started wetting the bed, having been dry since the age of three years, and has become extremely clingy to mother, often seeming unwilling to let her mother out of her sight. She views Stephanie's mother as coping well given the circumstances and as having good local family support. It seems Stephanie's mother is attempting to shield Stephanie from further distress by not talking about the death itself. Stephanie attended her father's funeral and has a memory box that her grandmother has helped her put together.

The health visitor agrees to continue her role as main support with some brief family work. She encourages Stephanie's mother to talk to Stephanie about her father's death. This allows Stephanie to voice her fear that: 'If daddy's heart was attacked then so could yours [be]'. It emerges that Stephanie believes her father was physically attacked. She therefore wants to keep her mother at home, where she will be safe, and also to keep an eye on her. Stephanie also mentions that she thinks she made daddy cross the day before he died, which might have led to his heart being attacked.

The health visitor explores with Stephanie's mother some age-appropriate ways to explain a heart attack: creating a story with drawings that Stephanie is able to construct with mother's prompting. Stephanie's mother tells her very firmly that she is not to blame in any way for her father's death.

The primary child and adolescent mental health worker also liaises with the educational welfare officer and school staff in exploring how they can help. It is agreed that:

- a member of school staff will meet Stephanie at the school gate on arrival each day to make it easier for her to separate from her mother
- staff will understand any distress or infantile behaviour and support Stephanie through this, if necessary allowing her to spend some time in the library when she finds lessons too much
- a key member of staff will be identified whom Stephanie or her mother can contact when needed.

BOX 10.5 Key components of professional support for the grieving process

Explanation about the terminal illness or death
Permission to express feelings or facilitation to do so
Reassurance about the normality of the feelings
Developing ways of saying goodbye

RESOURCES

Books for parents

- Kroen W. *Helping Children Cope with the Loss of a Loved One: a guide for grownups.* Minneapolis, MN: Free Spirit Publishing; 1996.
  This book is for parents of grieving children. It gives clear practical advice on helping children through the grieving process across the age range of three to 16 years. It explores the grief process and aims to help parents recognise how coping with death is an important part of a child's life.
- Wilkinson T, Rowe G. *The Death of a Child: a book for families.* London: Jonathan Cape; 1991.
  This book aims to help both adults and children to cope with the death of a child.

Self-help books for children and their parents

- Hollins S, Sireling L. *When Mum Died*. 3rd ed. London: Gaskell (Royal College of Psychiatrists); 2004.
- Hollins S, Sireling L. *When Dad Died*. 3rd ed. London: Gaskell (Royal College of Psychiatrists); 2004.
  These two books for young people aged five to 16 years explore in simple language the emotions resulting from the death of a parent.
- Mellonie B. *Lifetimes: the beautiful way to explain death to children*. London: Bantam Books; 1998.
  This is a simple yet moving way of helping preschool children understand and cope with death. There is a beginning and an ending to everything that is alive. In-between there is lifetime. It is the same for people as it is for plants, animals and insects.
- Mood P, Whittaker L. *Finding a Way Through When Someone Close has Died: what it feels like and what you can do to help yourself; a workbook by young people for young people*. London: Jessica Kingsley; 2001.
  A unique interactive workbook written for young people aged six to 16 years by children who have lost a loved one. Offers advice on the practical and emotional upheaval bereavement may bring and provides a list of helpful agencies for further support.
- Perkins G, Morris L. *Remembering my Brother*. London: A&C Black; 1996.
- Perkins G, Morris L. *Remembering Mum*. London: A&C Black; 1996.
  These two books, with photographs of the real people who have died, aim to show the importance of talking about grief and loss and remembering with love someone important who has died.
- Rosen M, Blake Q. *Michael Rosen's Sad Book*. London: Walker; 2008.
  Intuitive illustrations supplement a sparse text about the first author's grief for his son.

Fictional books for children

- Burningham J. *Granpa*. London: Red Fox; 2003.
  This book for preschool children describes Granpa nursing his granddaughter's dolls, mistaking her strawberry-flavoured ice-cream for chocolate, and falling in with her imaginary plans to captain a ship to Africa.
- Connolly M, Manahan R. *It Isn't Easy*. Oxford: Oxford University Press; 1999.
  This book for children aged four years and over tells the story of a child after his brother is killed in an accident. It follows him and his parents through their reactions, their feelings of sadness and anger and pain, and shows how they begin to come to terms with what has happened.
- dePaola T. *Nana Upstairs and Nana Downstairs*. London: Putnam; 2000.
  This book for four to eight year olds describes the relationship of a four year old to his grandmother downstairs and his great-grandmother upstairs. When his mother tells him that Nana Upstairs won't be there anymore, Tommy must struggle with saying goodbye to someone he loves.
- Hughes S. *Alfie and the Birthday Surprise*. London: Red Fox; 2009.
  Alfie's neighbour is sad about the death of his cat, so Alfie helps prepare a party to cheer him up.
- Limb S, Munoz C. *Come Back, Grandma*. London: Red Fox; 1995.
  For three to eight years. This generously illustrated book portrays the special relationship

between a girl and her grandmother. The girl grieves when her grandma dies, but then has a baby who looks and acts just like her.
- Simmonds P. *Fred*. London: Red Fox; 1998.
  This book for four to eight year olds explores the death and life of an adored family cat.
- Varley S. *Badger's Parting Gifts*. London: Picture Lions; 1992.
  This book for preschool children tells the story of old badger's death. His friends realize all the things he has given them during his life and take comfort in using them to remember him.
- Wilson J, Sharratt N. *Vicky Angel*. London: Yearling; 2007.
  This novel for children aged about nine to 11 years tells about what happens to one of two best friends when the other dies.

For those bereaved by suicide and other traumatic deaths
- Heegaard M. *When Something Terrible Happens: children can learn to cope with grief (drawing out feelings)*. West Virginia: Woodland Press; 1991.
  This is a workbook for children aged nine to 12 years to help them put into drawings their experience of trauma or death.
- Help is at hand: a resource for people bereaved by suicide and other sudden, traumatic death.
  This can be downloaded from http://webarchive.nationalarchives.gov.uk/+/www.dh.gov.uk/en/Publicationsandstatistics/Publications/PublicationsPolicyAndGuidance/DH_4139006 or www.cpft.nhs.uk/LinkClick.aspx?fileticket=xqL0EYfe%2FNA%3D&tabid=830&mid=1729&language=en-US

Agencies
- **CRUSE** can offer advice and support to parents/carers through their helpline or local branches. In some areas they may have trained counsellors who can work with children. They can provide information for families and also training and education for professionals. www.crusebereavementcare.org.uk
- **Winston's Wish** aims to help bereaved children and their families by offering: information and education; opportunities to meet other bereaved children and families; specialist support when grief is complicated; and training and consultation for professionals. www.winstonswish.org.uk

REFERENCES
1 Piaget J. Piaget's theory. In: Mussen PH, editor. *Carmichael's Manual of Child Psychology (Volume 1)*. New York, NY: Wiley; 1970. p. 703–32.
2 Kubler-Ross E. *On Death and Dying*. Routledge: London; 1973.
3 Worden JW. *Grief Counselling and Grief Therapy: a handbook for the mental health practitioner*. 2nd ed. Routledge: London; 1991.
4 Stroebe MS, Schut H. The dual process model of coping with bereavement: rationale and description. *Death Studies*. 1999; **23**: 197–224.
5 Goodyer IM, Herbert J, Tamplin A, *et al*. Recent life events, cortisol, dehydroepiandrosterone and the onset of major depression in high-risk adolescents. *Br J Psychiatry*. 2000; **177**: 499–504.
6 Hawton K, Simkin S, Rees S. Help is at hand for people bereaved by suicide and other traumatic death. *The Psychiatrist*. 2008; **32**: 309–11.
7 Her Majesty's Government. *The Children Act 1989*. London: Her Majesty's Stationery Office; 1989.

CHAPTER 11

Effects of parental mental illness (including substance misuse) on children and families

INTRODUCTION

Any form of mental health problem impacts upon not only the affected person herself, but also other family members and anyone else she lives with. There may be a tendency within some adult mental health teams to focus on the adult patient alone, to the exclusion of partners and children – or to assume that because the prognosis for the adult's disorder is good there is no reason why she should not care for her children. Of women with serious mental illness, over 50% have children under the age of 16 years, not necessarily living with them. About 25% have children living with them, often preschoolers.[1] Milder degrees of anxiety and depression are more common, and have lesser, but nevertheless significant, effects on the children. Similarly, children may be affected by parental substance misuse (including alcohol), especially if this leads to unavailability and neglect, or domestic violence (*see* Chapter 12 on Child Abuse and Safeguarding). Parents may be genuinely concerned about their children's welfare but unable to behave in a way that consistently meets the children's needs.

Children often cope well when a parent is ill for a limited time, especially if they can be helped to accept that their parent is *unwell* (implying recovery). The outcome for the children seems to depend at least partly on how well attachments have developed before the onset of illness, and partly on the quality of attachments with other adults, and how available these adults can be as alternative carers during relapses. The treatability of a parent's mental illness also has an impact on the outcome for children. A temporary period of foster care may be necessary in severe cases, if other members of the family cannot look after the children. Multiple episodes of illness may be more difficult for children to tolerate. Children may experience a parent's mental illness in a variety of ways (*see* Box 11.1).

Aetiology

Conceptually, it may be helpful to think of three ways in which parental mental illness and child disturbance may be connected.[2]

➤ There may be a ***direct impact*** of the parental disorder on the child.

➤ There may be an ***indirect impact*** on the child mediated by interaction or relationships, in particular the type of parenting.

➤ The association may be due to ***common factors*** affecting both parent and child, such as social adversity or genetic factors.

BOX 11.1 How a child may be affected by a parent's mental illness or substance misuse

---

Direct impact
- Finding a parent unrousable and not knowing what to do, or having to summon help
- Seeing a parent using drugs and not knowing what to make of this, or worrying about this, or disliking the consequences
- Not having any explanation of what is happening (such as doctors, ambulances, police, social workers or other professionals coming round). An explanation such as 'Mummy is ill' can merely lead to a host of further unanswered questions
- Finding a parent in a strange unfriendly place that doesn't look like a hospital
- Effects due to the symptoms of parental disorder, such as change of personality, irritability, aggression, withdrawal or bizarre ideas and actions
- Being distracted or withdrawn at school and unable to concentrate

Indirect impact
- Being left to his own devices excessively
- Feeling frightened or insecure. Not understanding the fluctuations in a parent's behaviour, especially if unpredictable or marked by changes and inconsistency
- Having to look after himself, or his siblings, or the parent – becoming a 'parentified' child
- Not being taken to school regularly
- Being embarrassed or frightened by his parent's behaviour and other people's reactions
- Experiencing inconsistency in his parent's behaviour and responses to him

Common factors – shared environment or genes
- Due to the effect of the parent's problems on the home environment such as marital discord and deterioration in living standards and lifestyle
- Having contact with a lot of strange people (involved in drug use), some of whom may be abusive in a variety of ways
- Exposure to domestic violence
- Worrying about developing mental illness or being in some unhealthy way similar to his parent when he grows up

BOX 11.2 Case Example

A mother says to a professional about her children: 'They don't know anything about my drug use' while one of her preschool children plays with a teddy and toy syringe, injecting the teddy.

BOX 11.3 Case Example

Walter is 12 years old when his father suffers his first manic episode – staying up for most of several consecutive nights, visiting exotic places with his latest girlfriend, and spending lots of money. Walter's mother, Victoria, seeks help from the primary mental health worker, saying that she thinks Walter is more affected than his elder brother Nigel, aged 14 years.

At the first appointment, the primary mental health worker meets with Victoria alone, at her request. They discuss the emotional impact on both boys, and practical considerations, such as how to preserve the family's finances and how to manage contact. Victoria agrees to bring Walter to the next appointment.

Walter, however, refuses to attend, saying that he would rather get on with things his own way. Victoria continues to come to appointments at gradually increasing intervals, finding the professional support very useful.

BOX 11.4 Case Example

Staff at a nursery school want to share their worries about Elaine, a 29-year-old single mother with a three-year-old son, John, at the nursery school. John's elder sister Jenny, aged seven years, attends the school most closely linked with the nursery. They alert the relevant health visitor about their concerns that Elaine has become increasingly unkempt in appearance and that John is constantly hungry, saying he hasn't been fed. The health visitor decides to visit Elaine at home.

The house has become less tidy since her last visit. Elaine seems rather distracted. She tells the health visitor that she was raped by an acquaintance three months ago, and that she is sure the neighbours are trying to take control of her thoughts about this incident. The health visitor asks Elaine whether she would agree to see a psychiatrist or a community psychiatric nurse, but Elaine refuses.

The health visitor asks one of her general practitioner colleagues to visit. He looks up Elaine's notes and finds that she saw a child psychiatrist when she was 16 years old who diagnosed depression with psychotic features and treated her successfully with fluoxetine. Elaine has had no involvement with mental health services since then. When the general practitioner visits with the health visitor, Elaine tells them more about feeling controlled by the neighbours and hearing voices through the walls of her flat. She again refuses to see a psychiatrist, saying that they are all mad and cannot help her: they don't listen, and all they will do is give her horrible drugs to take.

The general practitioner is jointly concerned about Elaine's worsening psychotic symptoms and the potential impact on her care of the children. He arranges a Mental Health Act assessment with the duty consultant psychiatrist and approved mental health practitioner. Faced with the prospect of a compulsory admission, Elaine agrees to a voluntary admission to the local psychiatric hospital, but only once someone can be found to care for her children.

This is more difficult than it sounds, as the father of both children lives on the other side of the country and Elaine does not have a recent phone number. He is eventually contacted the following day, when he says he is not in a position to look after both of them, and he thinks they should stay at the same school and nursery if possible. Elaine's parents are both deceased. When Jenny and John are asked, Jenny says she would like to stay somewhere close to her school and wants John to be with her. She suggests they ask the mummy of her cousin Philippa, who attends the same school. It turns out that this mother is the father's sister, and she is prepared to take both children on a short-term basis.

After a month's admission, Elaine is discharged with a package of care and support. The health visitor is invited to the Care Programme Approach meetings before and after discharge, and establishes close links with Elaine's community psychiatric nurse. The community school nurse at Jenny's school is also involved in the care package. Although social services are aware of what is happening, they have not become directly involved, stating that their input is not required, since everyone is managing so well without them. John and Jenny are gradually returned to Elaine's care. She continues to cooperate with treatment.

ASSESSMENT

The main message here is to ***think about the children.*** It is worth bearing in mind the following points.

➤ Children can suffer **significant harm** from parental behaviour and mental health problems.

➤ Significant harm can affect a child due to **acts of omission** – such as neglect or poor supervision – as well as **acts of commission** – such as involvement in delusions or episodes of domestic violence (*see also* Chapter 12 on Child Abuse and Safeguarding).

➤ Ask what (if any) risk does this parent pose to her children because of her mental illness or associated difficulties?

➤ The risk of harm to a child depends much more upon ***parental behaviour*** than parental diagnosis. The children of non-psychotic parents (meaning those with less severe mental illness, personality disorder, social adversity, domestic violence, drug use or alcoholism) may often do worse than those with psychotic parents.

➤ *Parental substance misuse* is associated with all forms of child abuse, including fatal child abuse. It has also been linked with unexplained infant deaths. Depending on how much it affects lifestyle, it can have marked effects on the quality of the child's care.

➤ Mental health problems may lead a parent to neglect or maltreat their children – despite the **best of intentions**, and even though she may also care about them deeply and love them dearly. However much a parent may love her children, adequate care may be impossible during exacerbations of illness – and children may not always have access to satisfactory alternative care arrangements.

➤ Try to understand the situation from the **child's perspective**. This may be different from the views of parents or involved professionals.

➤ Some children and young people are extraordinarily **resilient**, while others are more **vulnerable** (*see also* Chapter 6 on Resilience and Risk). An individual child's vulnerability depends on a number of factors including:
  — age
  — whether attachment has been disrupted by what befalls a parent
  — support from other adults – in the nuclear family, extended family or neighbourhood
  — support from the child's friends
  — social aptitude
  — intelligence quotient
  — success at school.

➤ Who are the **other adults** in the household? Women with mental health problems may be vulnerable and form relationships with violent or abusive men. Such women, especially those who have themselves been sexually abused in childhood, may be targeted by men who are eager to gain intimate access to their children. (And don't forget that about 10% of child sexual abuse is perpetrated by women.)

➤ How much caring are the children doing for the parent?

➤ How much of the childcare is being done by elder siblings?

➤ Think about the parent-child interactions:
  — what does the parent feel towards each child?
  — are the parent-child interactions generally warm, attentive and nurturing?
  — or are the parent-child interactions cold, disinterested or coercive?
  — what is the parental style of discipline? How is she observed to handle each child? Does she ever feel out of control, angry or violent towards them?
  — would the parent go to anyone for help if she felt she was not managing? If so, whom? If not, does this mean the children are at increased risk?
  — do the children feature in any delusions? If so, could this present a risk to a child?
  — could the parent be depressed enough to consider killing her children as well as herself?

➤ Which professionals are doing what for this family already? Are they aware of the full extent of the difficulties? Is what they are doing effectively safeguarding the children?

There needs to be some assessment of the difficulties faced by the main carer, but this should not usually be the job of child mental health professionals, who need to focus more on the impact upon the children and the adequacy of parenting.[3] Although a full *assessment of parenting* should ideally be done by social care or adult mental health, it is important that someone in contact with the child begins to consider the questions above, summarised more briefly in Box 11.5 below: this may be for instance a health visitor, community school nurse, school teacher, educational welfare officer, pupil support worker or primary mental health worker.

BOX 11.5 Summary of effects on a child to consider in assessment

What happens to the children when their main carer is ill or in hospital?

Is there another adult who can take over the care of the children?

Is there another adult in the household who could present a risk to children?

What is the child's role in the family (in relation for instance to household chores and parenting tasks)?

What have you been able to understand of the relation between the main carer and each child?

Which professional agencies are involved with the family?

MANAGEMENT AND REFERRAL

All professionals should prioritise the *safety and well-being of the child*: confidentiality and loyalty to the parent may need to take second place. It may be more difficult for professionals working in adult mental health to see things this way, as they consider that their first priority is to their patient, the adult, but nevertheless, child protection and safety must always take priority.

For child mental health professionals who have some contact with the affected parent, it may be worth encouraging her to *focus on the child* and his needs. Sometimes this sort of discussion can have a positive effect on the parent's disorder – if only by motivating her to seek help for herself. If it becomes apparent that the parent is too affected by mental illness or substance misuse to consider her children's needs to a sufficient extent, then involvement of other agencies may become more essential.

Possible ways of helping include the following.

➤ Can you *involve other non-professionals* in safeguarding the children – members of the nuclear family, extended family or neighbourhood? This is a risky option if done in isolation, and probably needs to be discussed with professionals from other agencies to share the risks involved. However, if it works, it is likely to be preferable to some other inputs which the parent may experience as intrusive or as taking away her autonomy.

➤ Have you discussed the situation adequately with the *other professionals* who are already involved?

➤ The general practitioner, health visitor, or other members of the **Primary Care Team** may be key professionals, as they may be able to appreciate both the child and the adult perspective.

➤ Can you engage the parent in **improving her parenting** and making it more child-centred? If so, then practical measures may help, including a support network and advice on how to focus more effectively on the child, to meet his attachment needs as well as his material needs. A local family centre with multidisciplinary input may be able to take on this sort of task, or in areas where they are available, Sure Start,[4] Homestart[5] or Family Action[6] may be of help. Drop-in centres, nursery schools, parent and toddler groups, parenting groups and other voluntary agencies may all form part of a package of effective support for the parent and child.

➤ For older children, a local **young carers' group** may help. National organisations for children include: Children of Addicted Parents,[7] The National Association for Children of Alcoholics[8] or Alateen.[9]

➤ If they are not already involved, **referral to social care** may be necessary due to concern about risk (for safeguarding reasons), or for additional support of the sort just mentioned, or to facilitate other forms of local provision. Respite foster care may sometimes be helpful.

➤ Referral (or re-referral) to the local adult **Community Mental Health Team** or **drug and alcohol service** may be necessary.

➤ Referral to a **community paediatrician** may be necessary if there is concern about one or more children failing to thrive or suffering from infestations such as scabies or head lice.

➤ Consider maintaining some sort of long-term involvement, or a '**watching eye**' upon the situation, especially if there is a chronic problem such as parental substance misuse, schizophrenia or personality disorder. If you don't consider you are the right person to do this, then it may be worth discussing with the other child mental health professionals involved who might be best placed to monitor the situation from the point of view of the children.

BOX 11.6 Practice Points for dealing with parental mental illness

---

Think about the children first – but don't forget to think how you can help the parent(s).

Involvement of the primary care team, adult mental health services and social services may be necessary.

Try to combine efforts to improve the available support with continuing appraisal of the level of risk and the potential need for intervention on behalf of the children.

If in any doubt discuss the situation (if necessary in the abstract) with social services.

RESOURCES

Books for children

- Ironside V, Sharratt P. *The Wise Mouse.* London: Young Minds; 2003.
  A recording of this story read by Paul Whitehouse is available for free download at: www.youngminds.org.uk/children/the-wise-mouse (accessed 24 March 2011).
- Wilson J, Sharratt N. *The Illustrated Mum.* New York: Yearling (Random House); 2007.
  This is the story of two girls living in the wake of their mother's depression.

REFERENCES

1 Oates M. Patients as parents: the risk to children. *B J Psychiatry.* 1997; **170** (Suppl. 32): 22–7.
2 Murray L, Cooper P. Effects of postnatal depression on infant development. *Arch Dis Child.* 1977 Aug; **77**(2): 99–101.
3 Reder P, Duncan S. Lucey C. *Studies in the Assessment of Parenting.* London: Routledge; 2003.
4 www.education.gov.uk
5 www.family-action.org.uk
6 www.coap.co.uk
7 www.nacoa.org.uk
8 www.al-anonuk.org.uk/alateen
9 www.al-anonuk.org.uk/alateen

CHAPTER 12

Child abuse and safeguarding

INTRODUCTION

This chapter aims to provide an overview of some of the issues surrounding the *safeguarding* of children – also called *child protection*. It is not intended to be a comprehensive guide to the recognition and management of the different forms of abuse or the bewildering profusion of relevant guidance and legislation. The amount of information and expertise needed by any professional (or volunteer) depends upon her role and her sphere of work. But child protection is *everybody's business*, so anyone who comes into regular contact with children and young people should be familiar enough with the basic principles of safeguarding to know when to be worried about a child's well-being and what to do about any concerns – which does *not* mean leaving it for someone else to do!

BOX 12.1 Practice Points: safeguarding is everyone's business

Anyone working with children can become worried about a child's welfare or safety.
Those working with any adult who has children or cares for children may also become worried about the effects on a child of the adult's behaviour, mental health or parenting.
In both cases, this entails a responsibility to do something about the concerns.
Think about what is making you concerned and why.
Be aware of your organisation's policies and procedures for dealing with safeguarding concerns.
Make sure you know to whom you should talk or how to get advice if you have any concerns.

Safeguarding and promoting the welfare of children consists not only of preventing or removing significant harm but also encouraging the positive aspects of child care, by parents and others. One of the key documents concerning this topic, 'Working Together',[1] breaks this down into three components:

➤ protecting children from abuse or neglect
➤ preventing significant impairment of children's health or development

➤ ensuring that children are provided with safe and effective care and nurture – which should enable children to have optimum life chances and enter adult-hood successfully.

The ***report into the death of Victoria Climbié*** by Lord Laming highlights the need for not only individuals but also organisations to take safeguarding children seri-ously.[2] The many recommendations of this landmark report led to a plethora of government guidelines, including the following.

➤ ***Keeping Children Safe*** was the government's initial response to Lord Laming's report and the preceding reports into avoidable child deaths.[3]

➤ ***Every Child Matters*** has formed the basis for much local government reorgani-sation.[4] It establishes ***five outcomes*** identified by children themselves as being important components of well-being:
  — being healthy – enjoying good physical and mental health and pursuing a healthy lifestyle
  — staying safe – being protected from harm and neglect
  — enjoying and achieving – getting the most out of life and developing skills for adulthood
  — making a positive contribution – being constructively involved in the community
  — achieving economic well being – not being prevented from achieving one's full potential by poverty or other economic disadvantage.

➤ Early identification of any child who is not meeting at least one of these five outcomes could potentially forestall the development of problems requir-ing specialist input or child protection procedures. The mechanism for this has been developed as the ***Common Assessment Framework***, which should enable information to be systematically collected and shared – with paren-tal consent.[5] It has the added advantage of not duplicating assessment pro-cedures, so that the family does not have to answer the same questions on multiple occasions from different agencies. The shared multi-agency assess-ment should lead to the agreement of an action plan monitored by a lead professional.

➤ ***The Children Act 2004*** supplements the Children Act 1989, placing new duties on agencies to safeguard and promote the welfare of children, as well as reiter-ating the importance of trying to ascertain the wishes and feelings of the child and giving these due consideration.[6]

➤ Agencies and organisations are made up of individuals, so children will be adequately protected only if everyone within an organisation knows when and how to respond. '***What to do if you are worried a child is being abused***' gives step-by-step guidance to enable anyone to exercise her responsibility.[7]

➤ '***Information sharing: pocket guide***' and related publications address the con-cerns that many professionals have about breaking confidentiality.[8] *See also* Chapter 43 on Consent, Competence, Capacity and Confidentiality.

'Safeguarding' is a broader term than 'child protection', introduced to enable early concerns to be shared and lead to appropriate action, rather than waiting for the child to suffer significant harm. Figure 12.1 attempts to show in diagrammatic form how different approaches may be applicable at different levels of concern. Different agencies may have different thresholds for intervention or acceptance of a referral.

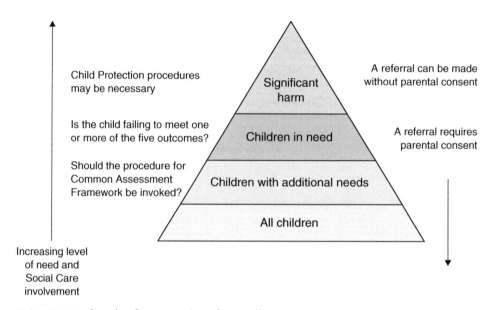

FIGURE 12.1 Levels of concern in safeguarding

BOX 12.2 Case Example

Tyrone is six years old when he starts to complain of a swollen toe in class. No one is very concerned about this, but his mother is informed.

Six weeks later, Tyrone's physical education teacher notices he has an ingrown toenail that looks as if it is becoming infected. Again Tyrone's mother is informed, but this time the head teacher strongly advises her to take Tyrone to his general practitioner.

A further five weeks pass, and Tyrone admits to his physical education teacher that his mother has not taken him to the doctor, and shows him a toe which is still red and swollen. The teacher consults with the school's safeguarding officer, who discusses the situation with the community school nurse, who is aware of other concerns about the family. They agree that a Common Assessment Framework meeting will be held to pool information and decide what action, if any, is necessary. Tyrone's mother agrees to sign the assessment that the community school nurse completes prior to this meeting.

What is child abuse?

Child abuse and neglect are forms of maltreatment of a child.[9] They may take two forms: commission and omission.

➤ *Commission*: someone inflicts harm on the child. Simple examples include hitting, making derogatory remarks or touching inappropriately. Categories of this sort of abuse include:
  — *emotional*
  — *physical*
  — *sexual*
  — *bullying*: sometimes included under emotional or physical abuse (*see* Chapter 22)
  — *fabricated or induced illness*: Sometimes in the past, this category was included under emotional or physical abuse: now it is more usually regarded as a separate category
  — *domestic violence*: It is important to establish whether the child is being physically abused or merely witnessing physical abuse, and whether the child is being emotionally abused directly or indirectly.

➤ *Omission*: someone fails to do something that could prevent harm or that is essential for the child's development. Examples include: not taking a child to the doctor when it is obviously necessary, as in the case example in Box 12.2; not sending a child to school; failing to feed a child; failing to sustain basic standards of hygiene at home; or not allowing the child to have any social contact. This falls mainly into the category of *neglect*, although the overlap with *emotional abuse* is often significant. The importance of neglect is that *it* is often neglected: it may be hidden from public view, and does not necessarily involve terrible things being done – merely obvious things that are *not* done: things that any reasonable parent would do (when healthy).

Both these forms of abuse are usually associated with some degree of emotional abuse. The abuse may be the responsibility of a parent, a carer, a relative, another child, a family friend, a babysitter, a trusted professional, an institution or – rarely – a stranger.

BOX 12.3 Case Example

Frank, aged seven years, and Juliet, aged five years, are removed from their biological parents and put into foster care when the police find them living in squalid conditions: a filthy house with floors covered in dog excrement. There has been concern at school for some time about the children's unkempt appearance and erratic attendance. There have been anonymous calls to social care about the children not being allowed out and being treated harshly when they do emerge from the house.

A comprehensive assessment including conversations with the children reveals that they have been abused in a variety of ways over a prolonged period. They have been locked in their bedroom without food. They have been beaten and bruised.

They have probably been sexually abused by adult relatives of their parents who have been sharing the house.

The children are initially placed together, but are then separated due to concern about joint sexual play. A prolonged series of court hearings eventually results in both children receiving Care Orders, and the court orders that contact with their biological parents should stop. Frank is too emotionally damaged and difficult to manage to be adopted so is placed in long-term foster care. Juliet is eventually adopted. Regular contact with each other is maintained.

The four main categories of abuse are now described, interspersed with case examples. We describe emotional abuse first, partly because is the most difficult to grasp clearly, and partly because it underlies most other forms of abuse. Please note that this is not intended to be an exhaustive account, but merely a summary of key features. The boy and girl described in Box 12.3 above were abused in all four ways.

Emotional abuse[10]

This consists of a relationship, rather than a single event or even a series of events, which makes it difficult to define and describe: it is particularly difficult to establish at what *threshold* safeguarding action should be taken.

➤ This is a pervasive pattern of interactions between child and carer, often beginning at an early age, such as:
  — hostility
  — harsh punishment
  — denigration (put-down comments)
  — rejection
  — scapegoating (blaming the child for whatever goes wrong).
➤ The child is perceived as deserving all of this.
➤ The carer may have inappropriate developmental expectations of the child.
➤ The child may be valued only insofar as she meets the carer's needs (an example is the teenage girl who has a baby so that there is at least someone who will love her).
➤ The parent may be unable to distinguish between the child's reality and the adult's beliefs and wishes (an example is the mother who was abused as a child who mixes up in her mind her abuser and her child – *see* Box 12.4).
➤ There may be exposure to inappropriate events, interactions or experiences, such as domestic violence, substance misuse or pornographic films.
➤ The child may witness or be made to participate in the exploitation of another person.
➤ There may be a failure to promote the child's socialisation:
  — by mixing with inappropriate adults, such as substance misusers
  — by isolating the child from other children
  — by avoiding opportunities such as nursery or school

- — by failing to provide adequate cognitive stimulation and opportunities for learning
- — by failing to contain or control the child's behaviour.
➤ Emotional abuse results in severe, persistent adverse effects on the child's emotional development.
➤ It is often combined with neglect, including emotional unavailability and unresponsiveness.
➤ It often occurs in association with physical or sexual abuse, but may occur on its own.

BOX 12.4 Case Example

Timothy, aged three years, lives with his single mother, Petunia. She admits to her health visitor that she thinks Timothy has violent impulses towards her. Petunia hints that she herself was physically and sexually abused as a child, but is reluctant to go into detail. She mentions how frightened she is of Timothy having sexual fantasies about her. She has not enrolled Timothy in any nursery.

The health visitor observes Petunia telling Timothy he is '. . . doing my head in'; that he is no good at anything; that it is all his fault they have to live in their awful flat; that it is because of him they never go to see anyone; and that she doesn't think she could ever love him.

The health visitor discusses the situation with a social work colleague who works in the local family centre, who agrees there is evidence of emotional abuse, but suggests beginning with a softly-softly approach. Although Petunia refuses to join any parent groups, she is eventually able to attend the family centre: initially when there is no one else there, then watching through a one-way screen as Timothy plays with other children, then gradually joining in with more of the communal activities.

Neglect
➤ This is the persistent failure to meet the child's basic physical needs:
- — food
- — shelter
- — warmth
- — clothing
- — cleanliness
- — protection from danger
- — access to appropriate medical care or treatment, as in the case example in Box 12.2 above.
➤ Neglect may involve abandonment or lack of adequate supervision – including the use of inappropriate caregivers.
➤ It is often combined with emotional abuse, including a failure to meet the child's emotional needs: the carer may be emotionally unavailable and unresponsive.
➤ It is likely to result in serious impairment of the child's health or development.

➤ Neglect may occur from birth or even before – for instance due to substance misuse.

➤ It is often neglected because the results tend to be hidden from view or overlooked.

BOX 12.5 Case Example

Jemima, aged seven years, is noted by her class teacher to be irregularly late for school, often seeming inattentive in class. Her clothes sometimes seem unwashed and smelly. Her single mother, Damita, seldom comes onto the school premises. The dinner ladies have observed that Jemima always asks for second helpings, as if she is constantly hungry.

The head teacher discusses Jemima with the community school nurse, who agrees to make some enquiries. The community school nurse knows that Damita has had mental health problems, but is not sure of their nature. She knows that the adult psychiatry team will refuse to talk to her about Damita, for reasons of confidentiality, although they would talk about Jemima. She asks the health visitor who used to know the family well if she has any information. The health visitor says she thinks Damita had a diagnosis of schizophrenia, but she offers to have an informal chat with the family general practitioner to get an update.

The health visitor comes back a few days later to say that Damita does indeed have a psychotic illness, which is sometimes more under control and sometimes not. At times she believes she is the bride of Christ, and then she is too preoccupied with the messages she is receiving to pay much attention to Jemima. Damita has regular visits from a community psychiatric nurse, and is on depot injections.

The community school nurse discusses all this with the head teacher, who in turn contacts social care for advice. It is agreed that the school will host a professionals' meeting rather than a Common Assessment Framework meeting, as they do not want to inform Damita of their rather vague concerns at this stage. The involved community psychiatric nurse from the Adult Community Mental Health team is invited, but does not attend.

Professional concerns escalate, leading eventually to a Child Protection Case Conference, attended by Damita but not her community psychiatric nurse. Jemima's name is put on the Child Protection Register under the category of Neglect, but all the professionals are reluctant to remove her from Damita's care, as Damita looks after Jemima very well when her mental health is in a good phase, and it is clear that Jemima dotes on her mother (in fact, Jemima probably looks after Damita far too much).

Various support services are put in place, with patchy success. At Damita's request (because she is terrified that Jemima will be removed) Adult Mental Health becomes more involved in multi-agency discussions. Jemima stays with Damita. After a year on the Child Protection Register, Jemima's name is removed, but staff at school continue to have concerns from time to time.

BOX 12.6 Case Example

Damien is six years old when professional concern arises about his single mother, Natasha's, use of alcohol. This results in Damien not always getting to school, although he appears to manage well once he is there, and seems usually to be well-dressed and well-fed. A social worker is allocated and decides to do unannounced home visits. Natasha seems nearly always to be suffering from the effects of alcohol, at whatever time of day the social worker visits. It emerges that Damien's father, who lives with his new partner, and Damien's paternal grandmother have been filling in the gaps in parental care. Natasha is referred to the adult substance misuse service, but is not able to keep more than a few of the offered appointments, and is unwilling to attend Alcoholics Anonymous.

Damien is placed in the Child Protection Register jointly under the categories of Neglect and Emotional Abuse. After many meetings of various sorts and the involvement of the court, Damien moves to live with his father and changes schools. He continues to see his mother for half of every alternate weekend. He appears to adapt well to his new circumstances.

Physical abuse

This is probably the easiest form of abuse to define and describe, and so is the most readily recognised, believed and acted upon. Examples include:
➤ hitting
➤ shaking
➤ throwing
➤ poisoning
➤ burning or scalding
➤ drowning
➤ suffocating
➤ fabricating or inducing illness
➤ anything else that causes physical harm.

BOX 12.7 Case Example

Katrina, aged six years, is changing for her physical education lesson when several bruises are noted by her teacher on her arm and side. Katrina says she fell when playing on a swing with her brother Gregory at the weekend.

Gregory's class teacher is able to ask him the same day about his version of what happened. He gives a very similar story. The head teacher and the school safeguarding officer take a close look at Katrina's bruises, and decide they are consistent with the story told by both siblings. Their mother picks them up from school and also confirms the same story. The swing is unsafe and the family are planning to take it to the rubbish dump.

No further action is taken.

BOX 12.8 Case Example

Ashok, aged five years, is taken by his class teacher to the local Casualty Department because he has a large bruise on his foot and cannot give any explanation of how it got there. The teacher persuades his mother to come with them after she has come to pick him up from school.

The paediatric specialist trainee undresses Ashok down to his underpants and examines him carefully. He inspects the foot. He takes a paper towel, partially soaks it in water from the tap, and wipes the 'bruise' off. It turns out to be grey felt-tip ink.

BOX 12.9 Case Example

At the age of 13 years, Jake is referred to the primary mental health worker because of concerns about poor school attendance. The primary mental health worker embarks on a series of home visits to try to understand what makes it difficult for Jake to get to school, and whether it would be appropriate to refer him to a tutorial unit.

During one of these home visits, Jake seems quieter than usual. The primary mental health worker will not let him play on his games console, but suggests he should do some drawing, without necessarily talking. While Jake is drawing, his mother reveals that his father visited the night before and was very cross about Jake not going to school. The primary mental health worker innocently tries a positive reframe of what feels an increasingly tense situation, and says: 'Oh, well, that shows that your father cares about you, doesn't it, Jake?' At this point, Jake erupts from his silence to say: 'No he fucking doesn't!'

Jake then reveals that, unbeknown to his mother, who was on her way to the chip shop at the time, Jake's father hit him hard with a belt three times in quick succession the night before. Jake reluctantly agrees to go to the local Accident and Emergency Department to get his bruises photographed, and social services become involved. This leads to the police interviewing Jake's father, who is so cross about the whole situation that he decides to stop all contact with Jake and Jake's mother.

Jake seems very pleased about this. It emerges that there has been domestic violence on and off for as long as Jake can remember – which his mother has not so far volunteered. She reluctantly confirms this: she appears to feel responsible for it, or at least for not adequately protecting Jake from it. The primary mental health worker wonders whether part of the reason for Jake's poor school attendance is that he was staying at home to protect his mother.

Jake has unfortunately missed too much time at secondary school for him to be prepared to go back there. He does however engage well with staff at the tutorial unit, and gradually becomes able to attend there regularly.

Sexual abuse

➤ This involves forcing or enticing a child to take part in sexual activities. It is not as easy to define as this makes it sound – there can be debate about what is and what is not abusive – so prevalence figures can vary a great deal.
➤ It can be divided into three categories:
  — penetrative – this includes vaginal, anal or oral penetration
  — non-penetrative, but with physical contact of a sexual nature (such as fondling genitalia or breasts)
  — non-contact activities, such as involving children in looking at sexual activity (live, online or on DVD).
➤ Sexual abuse includes the use of children in making pornographic photographs or films, which may then be shared via the Internet.
➤ It includes child prostitution.
➤ It may involve a preliminary phase of **grooming** of the victim by the perpetrator that involves the establishment of friendship and trust. Increasingly, this can be achieved via Internet chat rooms, social networking sites or messaging services.
➤ A proportion of child sexual abuse (perhaps about 10%) is thought to be perpetrated by females – who abuse boys more often than girls.
➤ Examples of situations in which sexual abuse may be difficult to define, or the boundary may be difficult to set, include the following.
  — **Sexualised play** may occur between children who are too young to give consent, but without any exploitative intent. This is usually associated with lack of adult supervision.
  — Penetrative sexual acts between **consenting adolescents** may be illegal without being abusive. In the UK, the law makes sexual activity involving an individual less than 16 years old illegal, although this is seldom enforced unless there is a clear difference in age or (more importantly) power. The law on consent to sexual activity varies between different countries: in Germany, for instance, the ability to consent to sexual relations is presumed to commence at the age of 14 years. The UK Sexual Offences Act 2003 makes it mandatory for any professional who becomes aware of sexual activity involving someone under the age of 13 years to report it,[11] but some professionals may wish to prioritise the child's needs (*see* Case Example in Box 46.6 of Chapter 46 on Sexualised Behaviour and Gender Issues).
  — According to the law, a sexual relationship between an adult female and a boy under 16 is held to be abusive. Arguably, a sexually mature boy of 14 or 15 years may be Gillick competent to give consent (*see* Chapter 43), and the power imbalance may not be as clear-cut as the law implies.
  — Is kissing involving the insertion of the tongue into another's mouth a form of penetrative sexual activity?
  — If an adolescent experiences an adult's gaze as lustful and intrusive, could this be construed as abusive?

BOX 12.10 Case Example

Irate parents bring their seven-year-old high-functioning autistic boy, Christopher, to their general practitioner, saying he has been sexually abused by the neighbours' daughter. The general practitioner is aware that there have been difficulties between Christopher's parents, who are now living separately, and that the street Christopher lives in with his mother and two sisters is a deprived area, with disputes between neighbours quite likely. He does not know the family that Christopher's parents are now complaining about, but one of his partners does.

The general practitioner asks to talk to Christopher on his own. After settling down with some drawing, Christopher explains in a matter-of-fact way that Jodie (aged eight years) 'sucked his willie' while they were playing in her house. One of Christopher's sisters was there. Christopher cannot say whether he agreed to this or not, but it seems he took his trousers off at the request of one of the girls. It is clear that there were no adults around at the time. The general practitioner explains that he will have to tell a social worker what Christopher has said, and his parents.

Christopher's parents are keen for the general practitioner to get social care involved: they themselves have not found social care much help in the past. The assessing social worker concludes that Christopher's vulnerability led him into a situation he did not understand, but that the whole episode was clearly an example of sexualised play. Christopher's parents are not impressed.

BOX 12.11 Case Example

Cynthia, aged 16 years, confides in her form tutor that she has been repeatedly raped by her stepfather. She is the youngest of three children, with two older brothers. She explains that her mother has known for some time about what has been happening, but has done nothing to stop it. She does not want to tell social services or the police. The form tutor admits very honestly to Cynthia that she feels out of her depth with this sort of information, and will have to consult with colleagues. Cynthia reluctantly agrees to this.

The form tutor discusses the situation with the school's safeguarding officer, who says that perhaps not much can be done if Cynthia refuses to cooperate, but in view of the severity of the allegations, social services must be informed. When contacted by phone, the duty social worker says she thinks they cannot do much. Then, having discussed it with her manager, the social worker visits the school to speak with Cynthia. To the form tutor's surprise, Cynthia agrees to see the social worker. Cynthia explains that her form tutor must have misunderstood her, and she has not been sexually abused.

Nothing more can be done – at present.

BOX 12.12 Case Example

A 14-year-old girl called Hanita has a rather poor relationship with her mother, and is in conflict about how much she can adopt Western customs: her parents were born in India. In particular, Hanita refuses to come home in the evening when she is told, but usually arrives half-an-hour later. On one particular Saturday evening, she is leaving a party later than she is supposed to, and has missed the lift with her friend's parents that she had agreed with her mother would be a safe way to get home.

As she is walking with another friend to the bus stop, a car stops with two teenage boys in it, who have also been to the party. They offer to give her a lift home, which Hanita agrees to. Her friend Felicity – a girl of 15 years – is more reluctant, but agrees to come along, mainly to ensure that Hanita gets home safely.

Instead of driving Hanita home, the boys take her to the empty flat of a friend of theirs, where they take it in turns to rape her, with Felicity looking helplessly on. The boys then drive off, leaving the two girls in the flat.

The girls eventually get to Hanita's home and tell her parents what has happened. After temporarily putting aside her upset, shame and fury, Hanita's mother manages to call the police and get Hanita examined by an appropriate forensic specialist – although this turns out to be surprisingly challenging in the early hours of a Sunday morning. Social workers become involved the following Monday.

Although there is DNA evidence and Felicity is a witness, albeit a very distressed one, the police have difficulty identifying the two boys. The girls know them only as John and Jeff, did not see them clearly in the dark, and did not think to write down the car number plate. The police enquire of the flat's owner, who says he does not know anyone called John or Jeff, but he did lose the keys to the flat within the last week: it is currently in-between tenants. The party's host tells the police there were a number of boys who gate-crashed her party whose names she did not know.

Hanita is referred to victim support for counselling. She attends one session, then will not go back. Hanita's mother gets a referral to specialist CAMHS, where she finds the support of a therapist with a Hindu background very helpful. Hanita, however, refuses to attend.

BOX 12.13 Case Example

A 13-year-old girl, Samantha, is admitted to the paediatric ward with an overdose of 16 paracetamol tablets. During her assessment the following day, she discloses that, a few days before, she got drunk and was raped by an 18-year-old boy.

The case eventually goes to court. The boy admits to having sexual intercourse, but says Samantha consented. The jury finds him guilty of unlawful sexual intercourse, but not guilty of rape, because Samantha was drunk at the time.

A fifth category of child abuse is worth considering separately, although it is rare. Children abused in this way often give rise to complex issues, and can occupy an immense amount of multi-agency professional time and concern.

Fabricated or induced illness[12]

➤ The carer may *fabricate* illness in a variety of ways, such as:
  — giving a misleading history – this may suggest a particular condition, which may at times be a mental health condition or a developmental disorder such as ADHD or autistic spectrum disorder
  — claiming the child has symptoms which are unverifiable unless observed directly, such as pain, frequency of passing urine, vomiting or fits – these claims may result in unnecessary investigations that may have their own potential for physical or psychological damage
  — falsifying hospitals records or charts
  — contaminating specimens of body fluids (for instance a mother putting her own blood in a child's urine)
  — obtaining specialist treatments or equipment for a child who does not require them
  — alleging abuse by a separated parent, as in the case example in Box 12.15.
➤ The carer may *induce* illness in a variety of ways, such as:
  — giving the child too much of a potentially harmful dietary substance such as salt
  — giving harmful medication
  — withholding prescribed medication
  — interfering with medical equipment such as infusion lines.
➤ suffocating the child – this may lead to fits or even death.

It is tempting to speculate on what makes a parent behave in this way, but dangerous to generalise. A mother may appear to thrive on the attention that accrues to her from the plethora of professionals involved through the child's illness; some may have definable mental health issues such as a personality disorder; others may obtain financial benefit. A psychiatric or psychological assessment of the carer may or may not help the safeguarding professionals understand what is going on, but a mother may refuse this or may find it difficult to open up when she is the one who feels accused. In some cases, it seems that the child may actually benefit from a false diagnosis of ADHD or autistic spectrum disorder if it enables the family to receive a much-needed boost to family income through Disability Living Allowance, or some extra help for the child in school, although arguably it is unfair on the child to be burdened with a lifelong label. But in many of the other situations mentioned above, the child is exposed to significant harm, and clearly needs safeguarding.

BOX 12.14 Case Example

Clarissa, aged 10 years, is the adoptive daughter of her single mother, Vanessa, who is concerned that Clarissa is allergic to multiple foods. As a result, she has a very restricted diet, and is becoming malnourished.

Clarissa's paediatrician recommends food challenges in the safe environment of the paediatric ward. There is some difficulty setting these up, partly because Vanessa is not confident that the ward staff will be sufficiently alert to Clarissa's allergic reactions, which include vomiting, headaches and bizarre behaviour. But the admission eventually goes ahead, and shows that Clarissa does not react to any of the foods that have been excluded from her diet – except for cow's milk, which gives her diarrhoea, and Coca-Cola, which makes her hyperactive.

This leads the paediatrician to consider possible fabricated or induced illness, and he involves social services. He obtains the medical notes from previous hospitals, and summarises the past medical history. This reveals a sequence of multiple visits to various paediatric departments with a variety of complaints, not all substantiated by investigations. Vanessa has described Clarissa as suffering from cerebral palsy, but there is no record of this diagnosis ever having been made on Clarissa by a professional, although there is an occupational therapy report from three years ago confirming dyspraxia. Clarissa goes to a school for moderate learning difficulties, which appears to suit her well. Vanessa has obtained Disability Living Allowance for Clarissa, and has entered her for a variety of sports competitions for the disabled, most of which she has won.

At a strategy meeting, the large group of professionals by then involved decide that there is by now enough concern to hold a Child Protection Case Conference, which subsequently recommends that Clarissa's name should be put on the Child Protection Register. The meeting also recommends asking the local child psychiatrist to become involved. She sees Clarissa with her mother for an initial assessment, but Vanessa refuses to return for a further appointment, as she is upset that the child psychiatrist agrees with the recommendations of the case conference.

The child psychiatrist is also concerned about the likelihood of fabricated or induced illness, and as part of her assessment, she persuades Vanessa's general practitioner that the child protection concerns allow a breach of confidentiality with regard to Vanessa's medical notes. The general practitioner says he will talk to the child psychiatrist over the phone about the notes, but not send her copies. From this conversation, the child psychiatrist learns that Vanessa attended CAMHS when aged 13 years because of difficulties at school; she made an allegation that her father, who had recently left the family home, had sexually abused her over a number of years, but then retracted this allegation before a videotaped interview could be done. At the age of 19 years, Vanessa started training as a nurse, but dropped out of the course after six months, and has not subsequently had any sustained employment. The general practitioner is not aware of her having had a long-term partner of either sex.

The child psychiatrist thinks that these features in the maternal history are compatible with the diagnosis of fabricated or induced illness. She forms the impression that Vanessa might in some way be meeting her own needs by getting plentiful paediatric involvement for her adopted daughter. She is able to put this view in writing without divulging the sensitive details which pertain to Vanessa and not to Clarissa.

Clarissa remains on the Child Protection Register for six months, but is allowed to stay with Vanessa, as she seems to be functioning well at school. Clarissa begins to eat a varied and healthy diet, and gains weight adequately. She continues to win competitions for the disabled, but this is generally thought to be enhancing her self-esteem, rather than doing her any significant harm. Professional involvement dwindles after Clarissa's name comes off the Child Protection Register. Social care does not allow Vanessa to foster or adopt any more children, but their file on Clarissa is closed.

BOX 12.15 Case Example

Peter is a three-year-old boy whose parents separated when he was 18 months old. He has been spending alternate weekends with his father. His mother contacts social care to say that she is suspending Peter's contact with his father, as Peter has told her that he has been sexually abused. The situation becomes more complicated when both parents obtain their own solicitors, and a variety of professionals become involved in assessing Peter, including community paediatrics and CAMHS.

The local social care protocol disallows making videotaped individual interviews with any child under five years old, but Peter is seen on his own for assessment by a paediatrician and a play therapist. During these individual assessment sessions, he is asked open questions about what might have happened at his father's, and gives no indication that he is uncomfortable with the contact in any way. He never repeats to any other adult the allegation that he has allegedly made to his mother, and does not say anything of concern to adults with whom he has regular contact, such as his maternal grandparents or the staff at his nursery school. These nursery school staff report that Peter is very well behaved there and socially well integrated, and they have no concerns that his care (most of which is provided by his mother) is deficient in any way.

Peter's mother complains about her community paediatrician and child psychiatrist not taking her seriously, and seems to be at loggerheads with most of the professionals involved, at one stage including even her own solicitor. At a strategy meeting, it is decided that it is unlikely Peter has been sexually abused by his father. However, there is multi-professional concern that Peter's development is being avoidably impaired by:
a) his no longer seeing his father
b) the repeated investigation of the alleged sexual abuse that his mother continues to insist must have happened.

An initial Child Protection Case Conference is therefore called, and Peter's name is put on the Child Protection Register. An investigation by social care of father's situation suggests no cause for concern that he is maltreating his son in any way. Mother's solicitor advises her that if she desists in her complaints, social care are likely to leave her alone. She eventually does so. Peter's name is taken off the Child Protection Register at the first review conference: by then, contact between Peter and his father has been restored, and Peter's mother has stopped insisting that he has been sexually abused.

Risk factors for any form of abuse

Certain children are more likely to be abused than others, including the following.

➤ Disabled children are particularly at risk, and three to four times more likely to experience any form of abuse than the non-disabled.[13] Disabled children are also more likely to be looked after, which is another risk factor for abuse. Particular forms of disability that predispose to abuse include:
   — language difficulty – to the extent of not being able to recount what has happened believably
   — moderate or severe learning difficulties – for the same reason
   — physical handicap – the child cannot get away.

➤ Within a family, one child may be singled out for any form of abuse for reasons that are not always clear but may include temperament, gender, autistic features or other sources of vulnerability.

➤ Some children do not receive the love and attention they require at home, so may seek this elsewhere, making them vulnerable to abuse by strangers, family friends or members of the extended family. Indiscriminate affection towards an unknown professional can be a dramatic clinical sign of this sort of parental neglect.

Fatal abuse

Child abuse may result in the death of a child. Most often, this is in families who are not known to relevant agencies until it is too late. In a minority of cases, the deaths occur in children who are known to services, but the severity of the abuse has not been understood until it is too late. Such cases may cause media uproar and/or lead to public enquiries: examples include Kimberley Carlile, Jasmine Beckford, and Tyra Henry in the 1980s; Victoria Climbié in 2000; and Baby P (Peter Connelly) in 2007.

It is clearly everybody's business to contribute to the prevention of such deaths. Therefore all professionals should be aware of the issues that contribute to preventable child murder. Detailed advice for healthcare professionals on the early clinical features of child maltreatment can be found in a relevant guideline from the National Institute for Health and Clinical Excellence.[14] Analysis of serious case reviews has found several common factors in such cases, which we summarise as follows.

Child factors

➤ *Younger children* are most at risk: two-thirds of child abuse fatalities are under five years old and half are under one.

➤ *Low birth weight* is a factor in a third.

➤ Frequent *house moves* often result in confusion between different boroughs, and children not being known to relevant professionals.

➤ Several or many *missed appointments* for developmental check-ups or health problems.

Parent factors

➤ A history of **substance misuse** and/or **mental health problems** (*see* Chapter 11).

➤ Parents may appear co-operative and compliant. **Apparent parental co-operation** may convince professionals that the child is not at risk, stop them from questioning further, or lead to crucial physical examinations or investigations being omitted.

➤ **Physical assault** by a parent is the main cause of death, implying that it is important to be aware of domestic violence – in so far as this is divulged.

Professional factors[15,16]

➤ Professionals rightly consider that it is important to focus on parents' **strengths**, but this should not preclude awareness of parenting **weaknesses**, dangers and risks.

➤ Professionals may be **afraid** of visiting some families, due to anticipated violence from a parent or cohabitee, or in some cases fear of catching something infectious (in Victoria Climbié's case, scabies).

➤ Professionals may take a view about a family that is based on limited evidence (perhaps only the reported views of others) and then fail to alter this view when contradictory evidence becomes available. Continued **curiosity** is important – not only about the family but also about the basis for the views of others.

➤ There is sometimes a failure to focus on what it may be like to be a child in a particular family. Curiosity about **the child's point of view** is crucial, and can be addressed not only by a degree of imagination, but also by talking to the child alone – something remarkable for its absence in the case of Victoria Climbié.

➤ There may be inadequate awareness of **who is living in the family home**: this seems to have been a factor in the death of Peter Connelly.

➤ Social workers and other professionals may be readily overwhelmed by the **nature** of their work. This could be prevented by adequate supervision – time for reflection and sharing of what makes such families so difficult to work with, and how much they induce despair and hopelessness.

➤ Social workers and other professionals may be readily overwhelmed by the **volume** of work. This should be addressed by appropriate management – limiting the caseload of individual workers. Managers may find this impossible when there are funding issues and recruitment difficulties, most likely in the inner city areas where these families are likely to be concentrated. The employment of locum social workers as a substitute for permanent posts is both more costly and more dangerous: the professional has only just got to know the family when she moves on to another post.

➤ The **chaotic behaviour** of some families may be mirrored by the professional system behaving in a similarly dysfunctional way.

➤ Agencies and individual professionals may **fail to share** important information. Even when concerns are adequately documented, they may not be communicated to those who need to know them, and professionals may fail to copy letters, have relevant face-to-face discussions or attend meetings. At times, this lack of sharing is based on a concern about consent: this should be addressed by the emphasis in 'Every Child Matters' on communicating any level of concern. At other times, it seems to be related to other factors, such as mutual hostility between different professions, or thinking that child protection is someone else's business.

ASSESSMENT

First, decide **what is concerning you**, or what is making you worried. Is it something you saw? Is it something the child said? Is it a pattern of events? Is it an inconsistency in the story given? Even if you do not know the child or his parent well, you may still feel uneasy and detect that something is wrong. Sometimes, someone meeting the child and family for the first time can see things that are not apparent to those professionals who know the child well – especially if changes have occurred gradually over time.

Consider **discussing your concerns with the child and his family**, especially if they are known to you. You should try to do this unless there are good reasons not to.

➤ Reasons for *not* having such a discussion with a parent may include a fear that this may make the child more unsafe, or a request by the child not to do so.

➤ Reasons for *not* having such a discussion with a child may be due to his young age, or a lack of opportunity to see him alone.

Ask a parent if she has noticed a change in her child: this may lead her to tell you about her explanation for the change, or she may be as puzzled as you are about the child's current state. Ask the child about how he is feeling and behaving: this may enable him to say what is going on. Even if he does not say much, having a trusted adult listen to him and take him seriously is very important and may be a first step in helping him feel safe enough to go on to reveal a bit more, perhaps on a subsequent occasion. It is very important (something which your concern can make you forget) to **explain** at the end of your meeting with the child alone what you are going to do next, particularly in relation to:

➤ whom you are going to tell what

➤ what makes it your professional duty to do so

➤ how this might affect him.

If you have decided to discuss your concerns with another member of the family – guided at least in part by the age and wishes of the child – you may need to give the same sorts of explanations. Arrange **a means of keeping in contact**: either another meeting or, for an adolescent or adult family member, a telephone or texting or e-mail agreement. Flexibility in contact arrangements may be particularly important for a young person.

Discuss your concerns with your colleagues: a named safeguarding colleague, a peer doing a similar job, a line-manager or a supervisor. If you are not ready to make a referral to social services, you can discuss the situation initially without giving identifying details, to see if the duty social worker agrees that you have grounds for being concerned, and if so at what level. A teacher may need to discuss the situation with the school's designated safeguarding officer; a pupil support worker with an educational psychologist; a general practitioner with one of her colleagues; a hospital paediatrician with a community paediatrician; and so on.

Make a detailed record of what is worrying you and the ensuing discussions. Describe in as much detail as possible what you saw or heard that concerns you – ideally using **verbatim comments** recorded at the time or **observations** noted as soon as possible. A brief summary comment such as 'The mother appears to be emotionally abusing her son' will be of no use to anyone who subsequently wishes to review the evidence. Of much more use would be examples of the mother's speech, such as: 'You really are a waste of space!', or 'If you don't shut up and let me speak to the doctor, I'll smack you in the face!'

And observations of interactions, such as: 'Mother scowls at child and child appears upset. Mother does nothing to comfort him.'

If, for instance, the child has an unexplained or unusual bruise, make as accurate a drawing as possible: even though you may rightly consider this a job for a paediatrician, you cannot be sure whether or when the child will see a paediatrician – the parent may refuse to take him until it has faded. Record in as much detail as possible how the child explained the bruise, and the parent's explanation: slight differences may be important, as discrepancy suggests a cover-up or, in the child's case, protection of a parent or sibling. Inconsistencies between the accounts of different people – or within the account of a single person – are a cardinal feature of child abuse. Describe the demeanour of both child and parent(s). How do they respond to your questions? Is the explanation credible? Who was supervising the child when the alleged accident or incident occurred? Who normally looks after the child, and for which parts of the day? Is the parent appropriately concerned or distressed?

Further assessment will depend upon your role. For example a paediatrician may decide to carry out a full physical examination, X-rays and blood tests, whereas a general practitioner may do a physical examination only and refer on to his paediatric colleagues or the local Accident and Emergency department. A teacher may refer initially to social services or to the local hospital. Different agencies have different protocols and assessment tools to be used.

How does an abused child present?

Different forms of child abuse present in different ways, depending upon the age and developmental stage of the child. There is no single manifestation, so it helps to be aware of the myriad ways in which a child who has been abused may first present to a professional. These are summarised in the following bullet points.

It is worth emphasising two contrasting points. Firstly, there may be an innocent explanation for almost all these symptoms, so it would be a mistake to jump to the conclusion that some form of abuse has occurred on limited evidence. Secondly, the way in which abuse presents can vary tremendously: child sexual abuse, for instance, can present with *any* child mental health condition – so this list is by no means complete.

Physical symptoms at any age:
➤ repeated presentations to Accident and Emergency departments with a variety of alleged 'accidents'
➤ repeated presentations to the general practitioner with minor ailments
➤ vaginal bleeding or discharge
➤ recurrent abdominal pain.

Physical signs at any age:
➤ non-accidental injury: bruises, fractures, burns and others
➤ sexually transmitted infections.

Psychological symptoms at any age:
➤ aggressive or out-of-control behaviour
➤ low self-esteem or feelings of worthlessness
➤ hopelessness
➤ unhappiness
➤ anxiety – particularly if it seems out of proportion
➤ symptoms of post-traumatic stress disorder (*see* Chapter 37).

Up to three years of age:
➤ unusual attachment behaviour (*see* Chapter 7):
  — excessive clinginess, insecurity or fearfulness
  — indiscriminate affection
  — frozen watchfulness: the child appears too scared either to move away or tolerate the approach of an adult – including his carers.
➤ sleep problems (sometimes related to attachment issues, or fear of what might happen at night)
➤ failure to thrive
➤ repeated failure to attend routine child health surveillance developmental checks or for immunisations.

Three to seven years of age:
➤ problems socialising at nursery or infant school
➤ appearing to be unduly hungry at nursery or school
➤ wearing dirty, ragged or smelly clothes.

Middle childhood:
➤ running away from home
➤ poor attendance at school
➤ indiscriminate attempts at making friends
➤ unable to make close friends, so becoming isolated or unpopular

➤ showing difficulty in trusting adults or getting on with teachers
➤ persisting decline in school performance
➤ poor concentration and easy distractibility.

Adolescence:
➤ deliberate self-harm, often repeated
➤ eating disorders
➤ substance misuse
➤ pregnancy (for instance with mystery surrounding the father's identity)
➤ promiscuous, unsafe or indiscriminate sexual activity, which may start unusually early in comparison to the peer group
➤ escalating antisocial behaviour, resulting in exclusion from school or involvement of the police and criminal justice system
➤ relationships with peers may alternate between being over-close or idealised and being conflictual or fraught
➤ relationships with teachers may also vary from a good working relationship to a 'personality clash'
➤ school performance may start off satisfactorily in years seven and eight, then decline inexorably
➤ poor concentration and easy distractibility
➤ running away from home.

Other warning signs of the need for concern:
➤ the child is not registered with a general practice
➤ the child is not on any school roll
➤ the child is not attending the school where he is on roll, or has frequent days off with vague symptoms that the child does not mention when in school
➤ the child is (or all the children in the family are) recurrently late for school
➤ the school staff or other professionals become worried by the behaviour of carers, who may arrive at school inebriated or apparently 'stoned'
➤ the child is functioning as a young carer for another member of the family.

Any of these may be a *cause for concern* as a sign of the child's predicament or distress. In general, the child's situation at home tends to be shrouded in secrecy, but there are usually signs at school or in other contexts that something is not right. Occasionally, a child who is being abused, perhaps quite severely, may appear to have no problems at school or in his social life. This may occur if the child has a natural degree of resilience and ability to succeed (in academic work or sport) as a way of coping or trying to forget about the abuse. This is an example of the child's interaction with school or peers acting as a protective factor – at least temporarily (*see* Chapter 6 on Resilience and Risk).

As *child abuse is everyone's business*, anyone working with adults who have mental health or substance misuse problems must be aware of the potential effects on any child (*see* Chapter 11). Administrative and support staff also need training on and awareness of safeguarding, as they may observe worrying patterns of behaviour or signs of child abuse whilst the child is in the waiting area of the office or clinic.

All such professionals should at least consider at what level the risks to the child may lie:

➤ no apparent risk
➤ some concern
➤ considerable concern
➤ significant harm
➤ death.

... and then discuss with colleagues as appropriate.

MANAGEMENT

Discuss your worries with some of your colleagues, your line manager or a named safeguarding colleague. If you are at the stage of wanting to preserve confidentiality, this can be done without naming the family or child.

Do not *make excuses* for what is concerning you or *dismiss* your worries to the back of your mind or convince yourself that it must be *someone else's job* to deal with. You must put the *best interests of the child* first: think about what it would be like to be that child in the situation as you know it or suspect it. For instance, the cultural practices of a country of origin cannot be used as an excuse: parents who choose to live in the UK have to abide by British customs and British laws that apply to the upbringing of children.

Before you decide to *share your concerns* with authorities such as social services, the police or the National Society for the Prevention of Cruelty to Children, consider any protocols regarding the sharing of information that apply to you: colleagues and managers should be able to help you interpret these. Once you have decided to share your concerns, it is best practice to telephone first to discuss the situation, and then confirm what you have said in writing: sometimes this involves filling in a particular referral form. It is important to follow recommended procedures to safeguard children.

BOX 12.16 Practice Points in dealing with possible child abuse

Think carefully about what is making you concerned.
Make detailed notes of the information you have gathered and your observations.
Discuss your concerns with colleagues.
Be familiar with relevant protocols.
Inform the child and family before sharing your concerns – unless it is dangerous to do so.
Share information with safeguarding agencies according to recommended procedures – in general by telephone and then in writing.

BOX 12.17 Alarm Bells in safeguarding

Things a young person may say or do:
- 'I am worried that a friend of mine is being abused.' (*see* Case Example 43.13)
- 'I am scared of telling anyone anything more.'
- A child repeatedly showing reluctance to go home (for instance from school or from the paediatric ward).

Things a parent may say or do:
- a disparity between accounts from a parent and her child: for example, in relation to observed injuries or prescribed medication
- a parent being very reluctant for you to spend part of the assessment alone with the child
- a parent demanding to see the notes you have kept on her child.

Professional issues:
- a work colleague not acting upon information which you perceive puts a child at risk
- a teacher or other professional asking for details of what a child may have told you in confidence (when there are no concerns about safeguarding)
- keeping concerns to yourself when you suspect there may be a safeguarding issue and you are uncertain what to do: you need to discuss this with colleagues.

RESOURCES
A book for children
- Hindman J. *A Very Touching Book . . . for Little People and for Big People*. Oregon: AlexAndria Associates; 1983.
  This is a useful book for children and parents which approaches the topic of 'secret touching' sensitively.

Books for parents
- McKay M, Rogers PD, McKay J. *When Anger Hurts: quieting the storm within*. Oakland, CA: New Harbinger Publications; 2003.
  This book clears up misconceptions about anger, explains how to control it and discusses spouse and child abuse.
- Elliott M. *Keeping Safe: a practical guide to talking with children*. 4th ed. London: Hodder & Stoughton; 1994.
  This guide on talking with children tackles a whole range of issues from sexual abuse to bullying and teenage drug-taking.

Websites
- National Society for the Prevention of Cruelty to Children: www.nspcc.org.uk
- Young Minds: www.youngminds.org.uk
- ChildLine: 0800 1111; www.childline.org.uk
- Child Exploitation and Online Protection: www.ceop.police.uk and www.thinkuknow.co.uk

- 'Keeping children safe from sex offenders'. This leaflet aims to answer concerns parents may have about child sex offenders living in their community: www.homeoffice.gov.uk/documents/child-safe

Further reading for professionals

- Gilbert R, Widom CS, Browne K, *et al*. Child Maltreatment 1: Burden and consequences of child maltreatment in high-income countries. *Lancet.* 2009; **373**(9657): 68–81.
- Gilbert R, Kemp A, Thoburn J, *et al*. Child Maltreatment 2:. Recognising and responding to child maltreatment. *Lancet.* 2009; **373**(9658): 167–80.
- McMillan HL, Wathen CN, Barlow J, *et al*. Child Maltreatment 3: Interventions to prevent child maltreatment and associated impairment. *Lancet.* 2009; **373**(9659): 250–66.
- Prinz RJ, Sanders MR, Shapiro CJ, *et al*. Population-based prevention of child maltreatment: the U.S. Triple p system population trial. *Prev Sci.* 2009; **10**(1): 1–12.
- Reading R, Bissell S, Goldhagen J, *et al*. Child Maltreatment 4: Promotion of children's rights and prevention of child maltreatment. *Lancet.* 2009; **373**(9660): 332–43.

REFERENCES

1 Department of Children, Schools and Families. *Working Together to Safeguard Children: a guide to inter-agency working to safeguard and promote the welfare of children.* London: Department of Children, Schools and Families; 2006 (updated 2010). Available at: www.education.gov.uk/publications/standard/publicationdetail/page1/DCSF-00305-2010 (accessed 29 April 2011).

2 Department of Health. *The Victoria Climbié Inquiry Report.* London: Department of Health; 2003. Available at: www.dh.gov.uk/en/Publicationsandstatistics/Publications/PublicationsPolicyAndGuidance/DH_4008654 (accessed 25 March 2011).

3 Department of Health. *Keeping Children Safe: the government's response to the Victoria Climbié report and the joint chief inspectors' report safeguarding children.* London: Department of Health; 2003. Available at: www.dh.gov.uk/en/Publicationsandstatistics/Publications/PublicationsPolicyAndGuidance/DH_4071977 (accessed 25 March 2011).

4 Department of Children, Schools and Families. *Every Child Matters.* London: Department of Children, Schools and Families; 2003. Available at: www.dcsf.gov.uk/consultations/downloadableDocs/EveryChildMatters.pdf (accessed 25 March 2011).

5 Department of Children, Schools and Families. *Common Assessment Framework.* London: Department of Children, Schools and Families; 2006 (updated 2009). Available at: www.dcsf.gov.uk (accessed 25 March 2011).

6 HM Government. *The Children Act 2004.* London: HM Government; 2004. Available at: www.opsi.gov.uk/acts/acts2004/ukpga_20040031_en_1 (accessed 25 March 2011).

7 Department of Children, Schools and Families. *What to Do if You are Worried a Child is Being Abused.* London: Department of Children, Schools and Families; 2006. Available at: www.dcsf.gov.uk (accessed 25 March 2011).

8 Department of Children, Schools and Families. *Information Sharing: pocket guide.* London: Department of Children, Schools and Families; 2008. Available at: www.dcsf.gov.uk (accessed 25 March 2011).

9 Department of Children, Schools and Families, 2006/2010: *Working Together,* op. cit.

10 Glaser D. Emotional abuse and neglect (psychological maltreatment): a conceptual framework. *Child Abuse & Neglect.* 2002; **26**(6–7): 697–714.

11 HM Government. *The Sexual Offences Act 2003*. London: HM Government; 2003. Available at: www.opsi.gov.uk/Acts/acts2003/ukpga_20030042_en_1 (accessed 25 March 2011).

12 Department of Children, Schools and Families. *Safeguarding Children in whom Illness is Fabricated or Induced: supplementary guidance to Working Together to Safeguard Children*. London: Department of Children, Schools and Families; 2008. Available at: www.rcpch.ac.uk/doc.aspx?id_Resource=3716 (accessed 25 March 2011).

13 Sullivan P, Knutson J. Maltreatment and disabilities: a population-based epidemiological study. *Child Abuse & Neglect*. 2000; **24**(10): 1257–73.

14 National Institute for Health and Clinical Excellence. *Clinical Guideline Number 89: when to suspect child maltreatment*: London: NICE; 2009. Available at: www.nice.org.uk (accessed 25 March 2011).

15 Reder P, Duncan S, Gray M. *Beyond Blame: child abuse tragedies revisited*. London: Routledge; 1993.

16 Department of Health, 2003: *The Victoria Climbié Inquiry Report*, op. cit.

CHAPTER 13

Behaviour management

INTRODUCTION

Parents complain when their children do not behave as they expect: this may be because the child's behaviour is extreme, or because the parents' expectations are not met. It may be the mismatch between parental expectation and perception that prompts referral to a mental health professional; or the perception of others who come into contact with the child, such as staff at nursery or teachers at school.

A ***parent's own childhood***, particularly her own experiences of being parented and of education, will play a part in how she helps the child manage the challenges of relating to adults in authority (the same of course applies to fathers; the female pronoun is used for convenience). She is likely to model her parenting on the parenting she received (and to a lesser extent on the way adults at school treated her). This could influence:

➤ the frequency and style of her play with the child
➤ the extent to which she praises the child
➤ the ways in which she sets limits or enforces boundaries
➤ the rules she chooses to enforce
➤ the degree of respect she shows each child
➤ the balance between warmth and criticism, reward and punishment.

Child factors

It is tempting to think that a child's behaviour is solely a reflection of his parents' parenting style. This is far from the case. Different children within the same family may show behaviour that is easy or difficult to manage. Preadolescent girls are *in general* easier to manage than boys of the same age; this gender difference can reverse in adolescence. A child's ***temperament*** is a major influence on how easy he may be to manage (*see* Chapter 5). Any form of special need or disability, however subtle, is likely to make a child's behaviour more of a challenge – so it is important to keep a lookout for this. But whatever child factors, obvious or hidden, may be exacerbating a child's behaviour, the way a parent responds can help to improve the situation.

ASSESSMENT

Ask the questions shown in bullet points – not necessarily out loud. Some of these questions should be asked (of yourself or others) when the referral is received, whether in a meeting, by telephone or by letter, or when you are preparing for the first interview with the family, parent or child.

➤ Is the behaviour appropriate to chronological age?
➤ Is the behaviour appropriate to developmental age?

Preschool children aged three to five years are expected to be active and bois-terous, and to test imposed limits. They are likely to have difficulties occupying themselves, and need more adult attention than some parents are prepared to give. This means that they are likely to discover ways of getting adult attention, such as being naughty, resisting instructions, or persisting in demands. A child of this age who does *not* have tantrums could be regarded as abnormal. A child with develop-mental delay or learning difficulties is likely to display the behaviours expected of a younger child. Box 13.1 shows a case example of a child whose age-appropriate behaviour is initially construed as abnormal. Persistence of such problems for long after school entry, or marked severity before then, may indicate the combination of deviance and impairment that constitutes disorder (*see* Chapter 1).

BOX 13.1 Case Example

Amy's parents ask their general practitioner for a referral to specialist CAMHS for assessment of ADHD. Amy is four-and-a-half years old. The general practitioner, rather than make a decision immediately about referral, asks the parents if he can contact the school.

During the resulting telephone conversation, the reception class teacher explains that Amy has a July birthday, so is one of the youngest children in her year group, and relatively immature compared to the other pupils. She needs a lot of support from the classroom assistants: with this, she is making progress; without it, she would be wandering all over the classroom and unable to complete tasks. Amy is also reluctant to separate from her mother when left at school. They agree that all this behaviour is age-appropriate.

The general practitioner sees Amy's parents again to explain that further assess-ment is inappropriate at this stage, but that a referral could be considered if the same symptoms are still causing concern at school in 18 months' time.

➤ Who is this a problem for?
➤ Who is asking for help? (Is it for instance the person with the problem or some-one else?)
➤ What makes it enough of a problem for someone to ask for help?

For instance, a mother who is just coming out of an episode of postnatal depres-sion is likely to be less tolerant of her two year old's demanding behaviour than a mother who is satisfied with her part-time work and child-care arrangements. A head teacher who has recently arrived at a school and is trying to instil a firm behavioural regime may be less tolerant of a child's extreme behaviour than a head teacher whose priority is to keep all his pupils. A stepfather who has recently joined a family may be struggling to find the right balance between tolerance and firm discipline.

➤ What has made the behaviour a problem *now* rather than previously or later?

When taking a history of problem behaviours, it is always worth wondering why the person for whom they are a problem has not asked for help sooner, or waited longer. Often the answer tells you more about the family or the professional system around the family than it does about the behaviour or the child, but this information is usually important. Behaviour may be identified as the problem when something else is really the matter, as in the case example in Box 13.2.

BOX 13.2 Case Example

Richard is seven years old when his educational welfare officer contacts the primary mental health worker about his uncontrollable behaviour in school and poor school attendance. His mother has been keeping him off school for three to four days per week. When he is in school, Richard gets into trouble for throwing toys in the playground: on two occasions, he has been sent home in the morning for doing this. The educational welfare officer has visited the home, and Richard seems well. His mother says that she is worried about his tummy pains, and wants to keep an eye on him, but has not taken him to the general practitioner.

The primary mental health worker agrees to accompany the educational welfare officer to the next home visit, with mother's acceptance. They discover in the course of conversation that mother's sister has recently died of stomach cancer at the age of 40; the first symptoms were similar to the kind of tummy pain Richard has been describing. Richard admits he is worried that his mother might get something like his aunt had, and that he gets more worried about this when he is at school. When with his mother, he reports feeling all right, but says his tummy pains get worse if his mother sends him to school. The primary mental health worker talks to Richard about the way in which some people get a tummy ache when they are worried – and then worrying about the tummy ache can make it hurt more.

The primary mental health worker and educational welfare officer say they will visit again when they have discussed things with the school and Richard's general practitioner. They explain to the head teacher their hypothesis that Richard probably wants to go home to check his mother is all right, and has chanced on a behaviour that allows him to do this. The head teacher says that Richard has always been well-behaved in the classroom. She agrees that he will not be sent home if he misbehaves in the future, but kept in the quiet room. The primary mental health worker speaks to Richard's general practitioner, filling him in on the background. The general practitioner agrees to see Richard if his mother brings him, examine his tummy, and ensure there is nothing serious going on. He will also explain that cancer of the stomach is extremely unlikely to occur at the age of seven years.

The primary mental health worker and educational welfare officer then meet again with Richard's mother, this time in school with the head teacher. Richard's mother agrees to try to bring Richard to school every day, even if he complains of a tummy pain; she will reassure him (just once) that he will be able to manage once he gets there. Richard's mother agrees to take him to the general practitioner if she thinks he is ill. She agrees further that she will try not to keep Richard off school unless his general practitioner says there is a good enough reason for his not going to school.

Over the next six weeks, Richard's school attendance reaches 90%. He throws a toy in the playground the week after the meeting, but is kept on the school premises until the end of the school day. He does not do it again. He still occasionally complains of tummy pains, but his mother realises that if she ignores this, he stops complaining about it.

➤ What are some recent examples of the behaviours causing concern?

This can help with filling in an ABC chart (*see also* Chapter 17 on Tantrums, aggression and sibling rivalry):

Analysis of the information in this table suggests that either Richard is over-reacting to provocation or his behaviour is inadvertently being rewarded by being sent home – or both.

TABLE 13.1 An ABC diary, applied to case example in Box 13.2

Date, time, place	Antecedents	Behaviour	Consequences
School playground, Monday, 10.45 am	Being called a 'mummy's boy'	Threw a plastic tricycle that had been left outside by the nursery class at the child who had teased him: it missed, but hit the shoulder of another child, whose parent subsequently complained	Richard was sent home as soon as his mother could come to collect him
School playground, Thursday, 10.40 am	None observed	Threw a tennis ball that he had brought in from home, which hit the head of a child who had been nowhere near Richard	Richard was again sent home

The difficulty with obtaining such valuable, detailed descriptions is that getting this information in front of the child may expose him to a long list of negative descriptions of him and his behaviour, which is unlikely to encourage him to feel positive about himself. One alternative is to arrange a time with the parent alone; another is to adopt a *solution-focused approach*, in which discussion is limited to occasions when the behaviour is better than usual (*see* Chapter 8 on Family Issues). Finding out what the parents have done that works can be affirming for them, and may lead to the development of more solutions. Some parents, however, may need to be able to share with the professional how bad things are before they can look at exceptions.

➤ What are the family factors linked to the behaviour?
➤ Who spends most time with the child?
➤ Who does the child get on best with at home?

Draw a simple family tree – it is likely to save time in the end. Initially, you can just include those who are living at home, and any other parent figures or (half-) siblings. Subsequently you can add grandparents, pets and later still if necessary, aunts, uncles and cousins.

➤ What is the developmental history of the behaviour?
➤ Were there any problems during the pregnancy or at delivery?
➤ What was the baby's temperament at birth?
➤ Was there any postnatal depression?
➤ How did the behaviour begin?
➤ Was it linked to milestones?
➤ Was it linked to changes in the family?
➤ How was the child perceived at day care/nursery/school?
➤ How did the child separate from the main caregiver?
➤ How did the child begin to socialise with others of the same age?
➤ Has the parental concern about the child been shared by professionals?
➤ What was the understanding of other professionals about the behaviour?

It is worth looking at any links you can establish. Concerns during pregnancy or delivery can affect the subsequent mother-child relationship. A baby who cries and will not feed or sleep easily can stress any parent (*see* Chapter 5 on Temperament). Postnatal depression (*see* Chapter 14) may lead the mother to be less responsive, and the baby in turn to become more demanding. Behaviours that arouse concern may start with toddling; with the frustration of delayed speech or language; with the arrival of a new sibling; at a time of increased parental strife or domestic violence; around the time of parental separation (*see* Chapter 9); or in response to the death of a beloved grandparent or pet (*see* Chapter 10).
➤ How can you and the child's caregiver(s) get out of the 'blame frame'?

Emphasizing some of the less blaming factors can be a great help for parents, as they may feel more able to cope with something which they can join with you to fight against. This is called ***externalizing the problem***. Examples include intermittent deafness causing frustration and leading to bad behaviour; a difficult start to life for both mother and child, from which they both took some time to recover; and being born with a difficult temperament. The danger is that the child becomes even more scapegoated, so it is important to describe the problem in terms which make it no one's fault. You could say, for instance, how many parents with a first child who does not sleep, won't feed and cries all the time are scared to have another, but, if this is the second child, they realize how lucky they have been with the first. Describing the problem in a new light in this way is a form of ***reframing*** (*see* Chapter 8: Family Issues). Another example might be, if the child were very disruptive during the interview, to say how helpful this is as a demonstration of the sort of problem the parents have at home.

In the case example in Box 13.3, a mother and her health visitor find something to blame for her unsatisfactory relationship with her son: the postnatal depression from which the mother has recovered.

BOX 13.3 Case Example

Ashok's mother Salima tells her health visitor that she thinks she is failing as a mother because she is always shouting at him. Ashok has just had his second birthday. The health visitor is aware that Salima recovered from postnatal depression only about a year ago; Ashok is her first child. She discusses with Salima the way in which depression can make it difficult to attend to a child, and how children respond to this by learning ways of getting some sort of attention. Ashok seems to have learnt how to make Salima shout at him – and her shouting has become a habitual reward for him.

They discuss how to break this cycle. The health visitor helps Salima brainstorm how she could give Ashok more positive attention. Salima agrees to spend 10 minutes every day playing with Ashok, and to find every possible opportunity to praise him. He has just started one morning per week at nursery, and the health visitor persuades staff at the nursery to allow Ashok to build this up gradually to five mornings. The health visitor visits fortnightly for the next three months, and supports Salima in finding ways of playing, rewarding more positive behaviours and ignoring the behaviours that have previously made her shout (*see* below for specific techniques). Salima becomes much more confident about her mothering.

➤ What can you observe about the child's behaviour, or the young person's demeanour?
➤ What can you observe about the interaction between the child and you?
➤ What can you observe about the interaction between the child and accompanying adult(s)?

Observation is a very important part of the assessment, whether you see the child alone or only with a caregiver. There are many facets of observation to be considered, as suggested in Box 13.4.

BOX 13.4 Some things to look out for when observing a child (and parent)

Does the child appear happy or sad?
Does he appear secure with the parent, or distressed by potential separation?
Does he seem hyperactive?
How long is his attention span?
Does he interrupt his parent frequently?
Is the parent able to share her attention between child and interviewer?
How does the parent deal with the child's behaviour?
How does the child relate to you, the interviewer?
Is he shy, does he seem frightened, or does he engage easily?
Does he respond to attempts to play or joke?
How does he cope with answering questions?

➤ What has been tried already?
➤ What worked and what didn't work?

Identifying measures that have worked in the past can help guide what may be best to do in the future. If you try something that parents think they have tried before without success, you need to explain how it is different, or else it is likely to fail again. Many parents are discouraged when trying new techniques of managing a child's behaviour. They find the behaviour gets worse and give up the technique. It is helpful to warn parents that this is to be expected. An undesired behaviour will usually get more frequent before getting less frequent (the so-called '*extinction burst*'). For instance, the first time a parent tries to ignore a tantrum, it is likely to get louder or more desperate.

BOX 13.5 Summary of assessment components for problems presenting as behavioural

Who sees the behaviour as a problem?
Is the behaviour appropriate to circumstances?
Is it impairing the child's level of functioning?
Why now?
Some recent examples (perhaps with ABC chart)
Developmental history
Family history
Externalising the problem
Observation
What have caregivers already tried?

TABLE 13.2 Four-P grid applied to Case Example in Box 13.3

	Biological	Psychological	Social
Predisposing (Vulnerability factors)	Salima's postnatal depression	Salima's mother-in-law has always been rather critical of her	Salima does not have much support from relatives with parenting
Precipitating (Trigger factors)	Ashok at a developmental stage to be confrontational	Though recovered from postnatal depression, Salima still tends to blame herself	Salima seeing other mothers at nursery being calm with their children
Perpetuating (Maintaining factors)		Ashok gets attention most easily by doing something that makes Salima shout	Ashok and his mother spend most of their time together
Protective (Resilience)	Salima has recovered from her depression	Salima is willing to reflect and change Ashok is still very young, so his habits will not be hard to change	Salima is well-supported financially by her husband

Your assessment findings can be summarised by using the Four-P model (*see* Chapter 6 on Resilience and Risk). Table 13.2 does this for the case example in Box 13.3:

MANAGEMENT STRATEGIES
Behaviour management groups

Behaviour management can be taught to parents individually or in groups,[1] or parents can merely be asked to read a self-help book (such as one of those listed under Resources below). Well-evidenced and competently delivered parenting programmes can improve not only the child's behaviour but also the parents' mental health and emotional well-being. Parenting style really does make a difference: parents who combine high levels of parental warmth with high levels of supervision are more likely to have children at age five who are more confident, autonomous and empathic – whereas a 'disengaged' parenting style is associated with poorer outcomes for children.[2]

Techniques which can be taught to parents of preschool and younger primary school children include play, praise, tangible rewards, commands, ignoring, distraction and consequences. In what follows, we describe these techniques, based on the parent training model of Carolyn Webster-Stratton, developed in Seattle, USA.[3] These techniques are most suitable for children aged from three to eight years, but can be used for younger and older children. As children become older, directing treatment solely at parents is less likely to be sufficient. Treatments that include older children or adolescents, school interventions, or seeking an alternative peer group are beyond the scope of this book (but *see* Chapter 30 on Disorders of Conduct).

Other models include Mellow Parenting (developed in Bangor, Wales),[4] the Parents Plus Programme (developed in Dublin, Ireland)[5] and the Triple P – Positive Parenting Programme (developed in Australia).[6] Up-to-date information on parent training in the UK is provided by the National Academy for Parenting Research.[7] A more informal structure of support for parenting, in which parents can graduate to become trainers, is provided by the ParentLink Network.[8] Effective parenting programmes have been agreed to include the following components.[9]

➤ They should be structured and have a curriculum informed by principles of social-learning theory.
➤ The content should incorporate learning opportunities that reflect social-learning approaches, such as:
 — skills rehearsal and role play
 — watching recorded vignettes as triggers for discussion of alternative parenting strategies, and
 — preparation and review of homework.
➤ They should include relationship-enhancing strategies such as play and praise, and effective discipline strategies.
➤ They should offer sufficient sessions, with an optimum of 8–12, to maximise the possibility of participants deriving benefit.
➤ They should not be didactic, but should enable parents to identify their own parenting objectives.
➤ They should incorporate role play during sessions, as well as give homework to be undertaken between sessions, to achieve generalisation of newly rehearsed behaviours to the home situation.
➤ They should be delivered by appropriately trained and skilled facilitators who are supervised, have access to necessary ongoing professional development and are able to engage in a productive therapeutic alliance with parents.
➤ They should adhere to the programme developer's manual and employ all of the necessary materials to ensure consistent implementation of the programme.

The 'productive therapeutic alliance' referred to in the penultimate bullet point is particularly important. Parents are the experts on their own children, and on what techniques will and will not work with them. It is important to respect this, and for the professional to be collaborative rather than didactic. Another level to this is that parents may often be reminded of their childhood by discussion of parenting issues. They may well cast you in the role of a parent, and possibly see you as like one or both of their own parents. A useful way of thinking about this is to try to treat the parents you are helping in the same way that you hope they will treat their children: positively and with respect (*see* Figure 13.1).

Play and praise are given priority in parenting programmes for good reason: disciplinary strategies may fail if they are not set within a positive child-parent relationship. The more effectively this can be developed, the easier it will be to

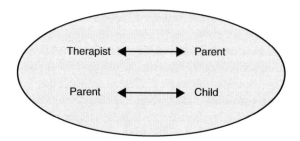

FIGURE 13.1 Relationship between parent and advisor in behavioural techniques

set limits and maintain boundaries. One danger of not prioritising the develop-ment of a positive parenting relationship is the ***positive reinforcement trap***, which occurs very commonly in clinical presentations (as in the case example in Box 13.3). This could also be called the ***punishment trap***. These traps are situations in which a parent neglects opportunities to praise good behaviour, and pays attention only to naughty behaviour resulting in lots of attention being given to the negative behaviour (*see* Figure 13.2).[10] The reprimands or punishments given for unwanted behaviour become rewarding to the child, so that the behaviours are maintained. For instance, if a child is ignored while playing quietly, but is told to shut up when-ever he whines, he is more likely to go on whining than to be quiet. If a child is constantly punished, she may get used to this, and seek punishment as a form of attention or reassurance. Hence negative consequences are much more likely to work if they are significantly outnumbered by positives, such as joint activities including play, praise, rewards and positive consequences (*see* below).

Another way in which unwanted behaviours may be maintained is the ***negative reinforcement trap*** (*see* Figure 13.3). Negative reinforcement is the rewarding of behaviour by omitting or ceasing a punishment or sanction. If a parent allows a child's whining to make them give up, and abandons attempts at setting limits, then the child will be more likely to whine again. If a child gives in and stops attention-seeking behaviour only when a parent becomes really angry, shouting or hitting, then the child's reaction will negatively reinforce the parent's coercive behaviour.

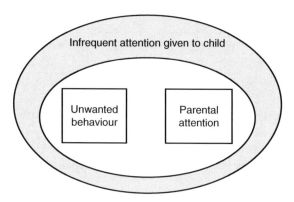

FIGURE 13.2 The positive reinforcement trap

It can be quite an effort for some parents to establish a positive relationship with a difficult child, and they may need professional help to do this. Parent(s) can be encouraged to make as much use as possible of play, praise and other rewards. The professional has to avoid the blame-frame: if she points out only what the parent is doing wrong, this will mirror the parent's management of the child. The task for the professional is to emphasize all the things that the parent is doing right, and praise effusively any little improvement in this, or attempts at new techniques, even if these are initially unsuccessful. This is surprisingly difficult to do – showing how difficult it must be for parents who are unused to doing this with their children.

Play
Professionals may assume that all parents intuitively know how to play with their children – but it is much easier for some than others. Those parents who as children experienced grown-ups as frequently and willingly playing with them will be likely to bring to their own parenting role a model of shared joyfulness with each child. Those parents who experienced as children little play or positive attention may expect their children in turn to play on their own and behave quietly, without necessarily receiving any adult input. Some children may be able to do this; others may need far more adult attention to be able to play or to behave well. This could be regarded as the second meaning of the phrase 'attention deficit': such children respond poorly to a shortage of positive adult input. In addition, some parents who have not received play may feel uncomfortable in some way about giving it.
The benefits of play for the child include developing the child's skills in:
➤ creativity and imagination
➤ vocabulary and general knowledge
➤ conflict resolution
➤ problem-solving skills
➤ the appreciation of values.

The benefits of play for each parent may include:
➤ developing a more positive relationship with the child
➤ the child becoming happier and therefore more fun to be with
➤ more compliant behaviour from the child
➤ more satisfaction and increased self-esteem from parenting tasks.

Playing with a child for 10 minutes each day is sufficient to engender such benefits. Techniques of play that can be taught include the following.
   Following the child's lead. It is important to allow the child to dictate the choice and pace of activity. Play may be the only time during the day when the child is in charge, and he will savour this; it may make it easier to accept the parent being in charge at other times. Some parents find it difficult at first to find an activity that interests the child. Once the child has realised that he has a wide choice and is in control, this will be easier. If parents are playing a competitive game, it may be best to let the child set some of the rules, rather than getting into a power struggle.

Allowing the child time. It is very tempting to take over or rush the child. This is not the best way to foster independence or self-esteem.

The value of attention. It is not essential to talk or join in the game, although this may help. Focusing and maintaining attention on the child is vital. Parents must not watch TV or read the paper while playing.

Descriptive commenting. This very un-British activity involves giving feedback to the child on what he is doing. This is surprisingly hard to do in a neutral way. It is tempting to ask questions, or even give a string of commands. It may help to think of this as like sports-casting. Providing a running commentary on children's activities gives them a sense of self-worth, and provides a foundation for labelled praise (*see* below).

Understanding the developmental level of the child. Developmentally appropriate toys or games should be available. Toys which are too young or games which are too difficult will not hold the child's attention. It is important to follow the cues given by the child as to what is or is not suitable.

Fostering the child's imagination. For play to be successful, a child's imagination should be respected, even if it means using a toy in a way different to what an adult would expect – such as using a building construction kit to make a giraffe, or using saucepans as drums. Imaginary companions are commonly involved in play (*see* Chapter 45). Make-believe is an important part of growing up, and play that involves fantasy can start as early as 18 months, progressing steadily into middle childhood, before beginning to disappear. It helps children develop a variety of cognitive, emotional and social skills. Fantasy helps children think symbolically, and distinguish between what is real and what is not. Role play can foster understanding of others' feelings. Examples of pretend play include using chairs and tables as houses and palaces, dressing up in old clothes, or using dolls or puppets to represent imaginary or real people.

Ignoring whining and yelling. Parents should try to get on with the play, rather than getting into disciplinary wrangles.

Preparing the child for the end of play. It is important for the parent's sake, and sometimes the other children's, to limit the amount of time spent playing. Ten minutes a day is enough to make a difference. Children are likely to complain when the play has to stop. This is likely to be less of a problem if a warning is given a few minutes before the end of play.

BOX 13.6 Practice Points for play

Aim to play with each child for 10 minutes each day.

Follow the child's lead.

Allow the child to set the rules – about how toys are used, or the rules of a game that you have made up together.

Watch silently, or pick out things the child is doing to comment on neutrally (descriptive commenting).

Warn the child a few minutes before the end of play.

The case example in Box 13.7 illustrates how only 10 minutes of play per day can be remarkably effective.

BOX 13.7 Case Example

Daniel is six years old when his single mother, Fiona, asks for help from the community school nurse, who in turn asks the Family Link worker to offer support to Fiona. Daniel has had a few problems in school, but Fiona says she is more worried about not being able to manage his behaviour at home, where he is the only child. Fiona says she cannot join a parenting group because of a timing clash with her work. The Family Link worker agrees to discuss some parenting ideas with Fiona over a number of sessions, following the 'Incredible Years' programme. In the first session, they agree to do a role-play about playing with Daniel: the worker plays Daniel while Fiona plays herself. The Family Link worker instructs Fiona to be as critical as possible the first time round, and then switch after about three minutes to being as positive as possible, using some of the techniques described above. Fiona realises how different the two extremes can be, especially when the Family Link worker describes in detail her (Daniel's) contrasting feelings in each half of the exercise.

At the beginning of the second session, Fiona describes how she has been able to play for 10 minutes every evening with Daniel, and how she has really begun to enjoy his company for the first time since he was a baby. Daniel seems a lot more content after each evening play session, and subsequently gets to sleep more easily. He also seems more inclined to do some of the things that Fiona asks him, although he still often gives her a hard time.

Praise

Many children appreciate a parent watching them in silence while they play (although some parents may find this difficult!). Comments and praise about what the child is doing may add to the benefit for the child, but questions and commands are less helpful, at least in the context of play. In any situation, it is helpful for the child to receive ***positive reinforcement*** for whatever he is doing right, and for any efforts in the right direction. One of the most powerful means of positive reinforcement is praise, which may have both verbal and non-verbal components. This improves the child's self-esteem, and helps her feel more positively about her caregivers.

Effective praising techniques include the following.

1. ***Selecting positive aspects of behaviour to attend to, rather than negatives***: For instance, 'I like the way you are playing quietly over there'. This is surprisingly difficult, particularly with children who have become highly skilled at getting attention by riling their parents.

2. ***Labelled praise***: This means specifying exactly what you are praising. It is much more effective to say, 'You've really made a good effort to eat up everything on your plate' than just vaguely, 'Good girl'.

3. Using **non-verbal signals** to enhance the effect of praise:
- ➤ tone of voice
- ➤ eye contact
- ➤ facial expression
- ➤ body position
- ➤ hugs or cuddles.

4. **Praising immediately** (within five to 10 seconds) – If parents leave praise too long, (depending on the age of the child), the child will not link the praise with what he has done, and so it will not be an effective positive reinforcement. (This applies to *any* form of positive reinforcement).

5. **Praising steps** in the right direction, rather than waiting for perfect results, or a complete task, before praising. This may also involve praising unsuccessful efforts. For instance: 'That's a really good try'. Another example: if you ask a reluctant child to tidy up, help him with the task and then praise him for joining you as soon as he picks something up.

BOX 13.8 Practice Points for praise

Catch your child being good.
Label what you like as you praise it: make sure the child knows what you are praising.
Praise immediately.
Use both words and signals (smiles, tone of voice, hugs or cuddles).
As well as praising complete success, praise attempts or partial efforts or small
  beginnings.

BOX 13.9 Continuation of Case Example in Box 13.7

In their third session, Fiona and the Family Link worker discuss different ways of praising Daniel. Fiona says she has always found it difficult to praise him, as he seems to resent it or be embarrassed by it, and sometimes even hits her! The Family Link worker asks Fiona what Daniel thinks he is good at. Fiona says he likes console games. The Family Link worker asks whether Fiona and Daniel ever play board games or card games together. Fiona thinks Daniel would find it difficult to lose, but she has never tried.

The Family Link worker suggests that before this Fiona might try finding things to praise in everyday life. She asks Fiona to keep a diary to show each time she praises Daniel and how he responds. Fiona's motto should be: 'Catch him being good'.

Fiona initially finds it very difficult to spot things she can genuinely praise Daniel about, but gradually finds more and more things, when she really looks hard. Fiona discovers she can praise little things, such as: Daniel picking up dirty clothes he has thrown on the floor, even if he doesn't immediately put them in the dirty-clothes basket; or Daniel opening the garden door for the dog; or Daniel putting the DVD player remote controller back in its regular place.

The fourth session is three weeks after the second, because of the Family Link worker's annual leave. Fiona reports that Daniel complained at first about Fiona's hugs and smiles, and seemed to feel that she couldn't possibly mean it when she pointed out how well he was doing things. But Daniel has eventually got used to Fiona being positive about him, and now seems to appreciate that she means what she says. He has begun doing more praiseworthy things.

Tangible reward systems

Unexpected rewards can be used to reward behaviour which parents want to happen more often. This means being on the look out for desirable behaviour, and thinking up appropriate rewards which are readily available. For instance, a child may tidy up his toys without being asked: a suitable positive reinforcement might be reading a favourite story for 10 minutes, straight away, or having a favourite dish for the next meal.

The 'when/then' rule: This means making a reward contingent on a behaviour. It is important that the reward is given after the behaviour, rather than before. For instance, '*When* you've tidied your toys away, *then* you can have a lolly from the freezer'.

The use of charts, stars, stickers and point systems: These require planning. Ask parents to write a list of all the behaviours they would like to see more of and all the behaviours they would like to see less of. The second list can easily be longer than the first, so some help may be needed to think of positive behaviours that can be encouraged. One of these may be the best one to start with. Define the behaviour carefully, so that it is clear what the child is expected to do. Then decide on a tangible reward. This could be a star or sticker on a chart, points that are written down, or poker chips which are collected. There may be a cash-in value when enough stars or points are amassed, either for a particularly desirable gift or activity or perhaps for extra pocket money.

For a successful reward programme, it is important to remember certain guidelines.

➤ Warn parents that such programmes are very hard work, and require attention to detail and perseverance.

➤ The child should be involved in planning the programme. This includes the choice of the most exciting sort of token (for instance, a particular brand of sticker), the choice of what they can be traded in for (such as going out to a friend's house, renting a DVD, or going to the cinema), and the precise behaviours to be rewarded (such as going to bed before a certain time, or doing one of a certain range of household chores).

➤ A reward is not a reward if it is given *before* the desired behaviour – when it becomes a **bribe** – and is less likely to ensure the desired behaviour happens.

➤ The tokens should be easily attainable at first, but the task should gradually become more difficult. It is best if the child can attain at least one reward each day.

➤ The tokens and rewards should gradually be replaced by social approval.
➤ The rewards should be inexpensive – or preferably free – such as extra time with dad in the park; a game of cards with the family or an extra bedtime story. The programme should be phased out after six to 12 weeks, and not continued indefinitely – although new programmes can be started.
➤ The programme should initially be simple, involving only one or two behaviours.
➤ Tokens/stickers/stars should be given immediately after the desired behaviour (not before, and not too long after). Behaviour must be closely monitored to make sure it is exactly what was wanted.
➤ Tokens/stickers/stars should not be removed for bad behaviour. This is likely to make the child lose interest in the programme.
➤ If the child has difficulty completing the set tasks, encourage the parent to be positive to the child, just as you should be positive to the parent. The child should be led to expect success, and if this proves too difficult, the tasks set should be made easier.
➤ The reward programme should be constantly monitored, and adapted to make it as effective as possible for the particular child.

Table 13.3 shows an example of a sticker chart for bedtimes and mornings.

TABLE 13.3 An example of a grid that could be used as a reward chart

Behaviour	Sun/ Mon	Mon/ Tues	Tues/ Wed	Wed/ Thurs	Thurs/ Fri	Fri/ Sat	Sat/ Sun
In bed by 8.30 pm							
Lights out by 9 pm							
Up by 7 am							
Dressed by 8 am							
Total stickers							

Rewards:

Daily	**Weekly**
2 stickers: a special snack on the way to school	10 stickers: a favourite comic
3 stickers: an extra bedtime story	15 stickers: a new DVD

Comments: The number of target behaviours in the chart, and the type and timing of rewards, will need to be adjusted to the individual child. Some children need all rewards straight away. Some can hold on to the idea of a reward for a whole day or a whole week. It is essential to adapt any tangible reward programme to the individual circumstances of parent and child.

BOX 13.10 Practice Points for rewards

You can add a reward to your praise when you catch your child being good.
You can promise a reward for certain behaviour – the 'When . . . then . . .' rule.
Give rewards immediately after the desired behaviour (not before and not too long after).
Make sure the child knows what each reward is for.
You can build a reward programme out of stars, stickers, tokens or points.

The following case example illustrates the need for attention to detail with reward programmes.

BOX 13.11 Case Example

The family support worker meets with Juliette for a review of progress with the reward chart they agreed a week ago. Juliette describes the absolute failure of her first week's attempts at using a sticker chart to change her son Mike's behaviour. Mike is four years old and has been receiving stickers for sitting at the dining table for his meals. Instead of sitting at the table, he repeatedly gets down and demands a sticker before he returns to the table. This is causing major arguments between mother and child: Juliette has resorted to removing stickers each time he argues with her. Juliette is frustrated, upset and uncomfortable about the impact her conflict with Mike is having on his two-year-old sister. The family support worker agrees to discuss Mike's problem with the primary mental health worker who is attached to the children's centre where she works – and then get back to Juliette.

The primary mental health worker listens carefully to the family support worker's description of what Juliette has been doing. She suggests that Juliette should be advised to renegotiate the sticker chart by explaining very clearly to Mike what he has to do to get a sticker. Mike should be allowed to choose the particular type of stickers to use. He will have to sit at the table for each meal and, if he gets down, return to his seat immediately when Juliette asks him. Juliette should be advised to keep mealtimes short to begin with, to make it easier for Mike to earn a sticker. It is important that Juliette should ensure Mike starts getting stickers, otherwise the reward programme won't get off the ground. Mike should not have stickers taken away. Juliette should try not to show her frustration or anger if Mike fails to comply at first. At every stage, Mike should be able to answer clearly when asked what he has to do to get a sticker. Attempts at getting a sticker when he hasn't done this are to be ignored, as are tantrums. Juliette should say she is sorry if Mike does not get a sticker, and suggest how he can get one next time. Juliette and Mike should agree on the number of stickers that will lead to a secondary reward, which should be inexpensive or even of no monetary value, such as some special time doing something Mike really likes. Once Mike has got into the habit of enjoying rewards, Juliette can renegotiate the behaviour he needs to show to get a sticker, and the number of stickers he needs to earn before he gets a secondary reward.

The family support worker gets back to Juliette and explains this new advice.

Two weeks later, Juliette reports a much happier situation. Mike has at last enjoyed getting a Batman sticker each time he sits for a mealtime: having earned three stickers in the first two days, he has been further rewarded with a promised trip to an airport perimeter fence to watch the aeroplanes taking off and landing. Mike is now enthusiastic about getting stickers. Juliette has recalibrated the reward programme so that Mike has to sit at the table slightly longer for each sticker, and has to earn five stickers for the next exchange reward, which will be a special trip to fly his kite. Juliette is now much happier, and can see how using this system of rewards helps to improve Mike's behaviour at mealtimes.

Effective commands

An *effective command* should be simple, developmentally appropriate, and mean something definite. 'Be good!' or 'Show me some respect!' are too vague, and do not specify to the child what he has to do. 'Please would you do what I say before I have finished counting to five' is more specific, but would have to be simplified for a young child (probably by breaking the statement down into small bits). Commands should also be positive and polite, and should use 'do' in preference to 'don't' or 'stop'. For instance: 'Please pick up that sweet paper'.

Commands which specify what should not be done are likely to encourage just that behaviour. This is because it is reminding the child of the very behaviour that the parent does not want him to do and therefore unintentionally cueing him to do it. For example, telling a young child 'Don't touch the television' actually draws his attention to the very thing that is to be left alone. Prior to this the child may not even have had the television in his thoughts. 'Come and play with this toy' is a much more effective command.

Commands are more effective if spoken in simple language, adapted to the child's developmental level. The parent must ensure she has the child's attention before speaking. The adult may need to crouch down so that faces are on the same level and eye contact is well-established.

Unclear commands are less effective. For instance, 'Your clothes are all over the floor of the bedroom' is not really a command at all, but a critical comment, which is likely to breed resentment rather than co-operative action. Better would be: 'Could you please put those clothes into the clothes cupboard?'

It is all too easy as a parent to shower your child with *multiple commands*. A child may get caught in a bewildering muddle of things he is expected to do, so it is small wonder he doesn't achieve most of them. It is much more effective to give only one command at a time. Some commands are smothered in a flurry of explanations or questions. Many children will argue with the explanation, so that the original command is forgotten. Help parents think about what they are asking, and prune commands to only those that are necessary, with the minimum of explanation, and no questions.

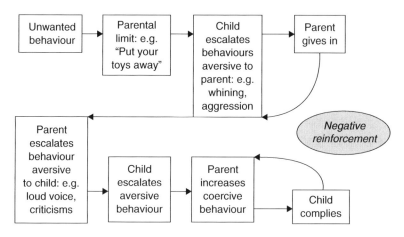

FIGURE 13.3 The negative reinforcement trap

This process may be helped by getting both parents to decide on a short list of essential **household rules**. These could be posted on the fridge, so that everyone, including babysitters, will know what the rules are.

Children should be given an opportunity to comply with a command. It is essential to '**catch them being good**', and praise compliance as soon as it appears, even if it is only partial: 'Thank you for putting your trousers away so neatly' (even though the other clothes have not been touched).

Alternatives to straight commands include a '**when/then**' **command**; for instance, 'When you have put the sweet papers in the bin, then you can go out and play with your friend' (*see* tangible reward systems above). This gives the child the option of not complying, but the phrasing anticipates compliance. A slightly different sort of instruction is an '**if/then**' **warning**, which specifies an undesirable consequence for non-compliance. For instance, 'If you don't close the door when you go outside, then you will have to go to time-out', or 'If you don't eat your food during the mealtime, then you won't be able to eat it later'. (*See* time out and logical consequences below.)

A command is more likely to be effective if the child is prepared for it. Interrupting an engrossing activity with an unwelcome instruction is unlikely to achieve much except aggravation. A **warning** could prepare the child: for instance, to a child who is busy building something with blocks, a parent could say: 'In two more minutes, it will be time to put the blocks away'. For children to whom 'two minutes' means nothing, a timer could be used. Warnings can be even more effective if they take into account children's wishes, for instance: 'When that television programme is finished, please come to the table for dinner'.

For children to whom more than one adult gives commands, it is important that **each supports the other**. This means being aware of the commands issued by the other adult, reinforcing compliance of these, and not issuing counter-commands.

Children will ignore commands if there is no **follow through.** For compliance, there should be reinforcement, in the form of praise or other reward. For non-compliance, parents need to decide whether they want to make an issue on this occasion; if for instance either child or parent is exhausted, then it may be safer simply to ignore. The danger of ignoring too often is that children learn they do not have to comply; the danger of following through with every non-compliant episode is that it may turn the relationship into a perpetual conflict. If the parent decides to follow through, this should be with either a consequence or with time-out (*see* below for more about consequences and time-out), after a warning statement such as: 'If you don't put the sweet papers in the bin instead of on the floor, you won't be able to watch your favourite programme'. Any consequence should be commensurate rather than excessive.

BOX 13.12 Practice Points for commands

Make sure the child understands what you want her to do.
Do you have the child's attention? (Eye contact? Faces on the same level?)
Keep commands simple.
If possible, give only one command at a time.
Be polite to your child and show her respect (as you would expect from her).
Give praise (or perhaps a reward) immediately the child complies.
To deal with non-compliance:
- ensure it matters (if it doesn't, ignore it)
- repeat the command (can you make it clearer and simpler?)
- warn of consequence or time-out
- wait to see if there is any move to comply: if there is (however small), praise it at once
- if it becomes clear that compliance is not coming, do what you have warned.

BOX 13.13 Continuation of Case Example in Boxes 13.7 and 13.9

In session five, the Family Link worker and Fiona discuss how Fiona could adjust the way she tells Daniel what to do. They role-play different ways of giving commands, again with the Family Link worker playing Daniel and Fiona playing herself. The Family Link worker asks Fiona to try first to give a command in a way that would be least likely to be successful, and then improve on it. Fiona stands with her side to Daniel, not looking at him but shouting at him to tidy his toys away. Daniel (the Family Link worker) just goes on playing.

In the replay, Fiona sits on the floor next to Daniel so that she is on a level with him and looking straight at him. She says, 'Please help me tidy your toys away'. Daniel stares at his mother, bemused. She continues: 'Where do you think we should put your Lego?' Daniel again looks rather puzzled. Fiona asks Daniel whether he wants to put the Lego in the toy tub or on his special shelf. He thinks for a bit, and then says he thinks it would go best in the toy tub, providing they keep everything else out of the tub. So Fiona starts putting the Lego in the tub. Daniel joins in. As soon as he puts the first piece in the tub, Fiona praises him non-verbally by giving him a hug (which is easy as they are already almost touching). She says: 'Thank you so much for helping me put your toys away'. Daniel appears to feel a bit awkward, but goes on helping Fiona tidy up.

Feeding back from the role-play, the Family Link worker observes that as Daniel she felt his views were being respected and he wasn't any longer just being told to do something. He didn't really feel as if he was complying with an instruction, but rather that Fiona was listening to what he wanted, and helping him do it. Fiona says that she felt much more in control, in spite of (or because of?) giving more control to Daniel.

Ignoring and distraction

Some parents think that ignoring is not a useful form of discipline. The truth is that it is not only a very powerful technique but also very difficult to carry out. Many children prefer to be screamed at than ignored. As shouting, or any other sort of attention, is likely to maintain unwanted behaviours, those which are not dangerous can often be eliminated if systematically ignored, especially if positive attention for desirable behaviour is given instead. Behaviours which can successfully be ignored in children include:

➤ whining
➤ temper tantrums
➤ protests when prohibited from doing or having something
➤ swearing
➤ facial grimaces
➤ minor squabbles between children
➤ nose-picking
➤ nail-biting
➤ brief crying in the middle of the night
➤ messy eating
➤ faddy eating.

Ignoring means avoiding all verbal and non-verbal communication with the child, and moving away, so as to avoid physical contact. The word 'ignoring' doesn't really do justice to this very hard bit of parenting, so it may be clearer to call it '*actively remaining neutral*' (even though this is a bit of a mouthful). It is best for the parent to avert gaze from the child, at an angle of 90–180°, so as to avoid inadvertent facial expressions, which either through annoyance or amusement, are reinforcing. The parent might do something unrelated, such as reading the paper. The parent should not express any anger, and should keep a neutral facial expression: the aim is to make the child think the adult is not affected at all by her behaviour. It may be helpful for the parent to explain ignoring to the child, but this should be done in advance, when the child is calm and receptive, not while she is doing something that requires ignoring.

Distraction works well in combination with ignoring. This can take two forms: the parent distracting the child onto an alternative activity, or the parent distracting herself so as not to give any attention to the child. The best time to introduce a distraction for a child is before she has started to wind up, or when she has started to calm down.

Tell parents of the expected '*extinction burst*': the rule is that the ignored behaviour will get worse before it gets better. Parents who expect this are less likely to see it as a sign of the technique not working and more likely to persist. For instance, a four-year-old girl wants to go outside, and argues with her mother about this for several minutes. Her mother decides to issue a firm command: 'I am afraid you cannot go outside at the moment, and that is final', and then ignores her daughter's protests. The girl escalates her demands in an effort to get what she wants. Providing the mother persists in ignoring the arguments, the girl will eventually stop, but not before becoming significantly more obnoxious, and trying to prolong things beyond the limit of her mother's patience. If the mother gives in, she will be negatively reinforcing the girl's arguing, whining and non-compliance. This is one reason why ignoring is so difficult to carry out.

Sometimes parents give up on ignoring or other behavioural interventions, such as time-out, because they feel they are **not working**. Looking more closely at what is happening may often reveal that the technique is actually starting to work. It may therefore be helpful for parents keep a **diary** of episodes that focuses on recording their success. For example, a record of the frequency and duration of temper outbursts may reveal that they increase initially after a new policy of ignoring is instituted, and then subside gradually. Parents' expectations often change with circumstances, so they may not notice gradual improvements without some sort of record. If, for instance, parents consistently apply the technique of actively remaining neutral, the record is likely to show the frequency and duration of the ignored behaviour diminishing over time. Such an account could be at least partly diagrammatic rather than exclusively based on words. Rather than simply instructing parents to keep a diary, it may be more effective to ask parents to think of how best to monitor success and keep track of it. This may lead a parent to suggest a diary or something equivalent: having suggested it herself, she is much more likely to see the benefits and persist with it.

Another difficulty some parents have with ignoring is that they feel it is *not punishing the child enough*. In fact it is more effective than punishment, because it maintains a positive relationship with the child and shows her that you are not affected by her actions or feelings. It is important, however, not to maintain ignoring over such a long period that it becomes a punishment or an expression of anger. It is most effective when followed immediately by giving positive attention for a desired behaviour, preferably within five seconds of this appearing.

It is tempting for the parent to **leave the room** in order to ignore more effectively. This can at times be very successful. The difficulty with it is not being available to witness the return of behaviours that can be positively reinforced. It can also make some children anxious. In more extreme cases, ignoring can be *abusive*, for instance threatening to leave or abandon the child, which is counterproductive, as it is a threat which should not be carried out, and makes the child feel insecure.

Ignoring can be effective in the presence of siblings if it involves differential praise, for instance at a meal time when the child who is eating quietly should be praised while the child who is throwing food around should be ignored. However, with other behaviours *attention from siblings or others* (for instance in a bus or supermarket) can make ignoring impossible. Ignoring is also not advisable for destructive behaviours, lying, stealing or forgetting agreed chores.

BOX 13.14 Practice Points for ignoring (actively remaining neutral) and distraction

Ignoring is much harder than doing nothing.
It involves not letting yourself get uptight about something your child is doing.
If you find it difficult not to get irritated, find a distraction for yourself.
Ignoring requires some planning: for instance, what can you choose to ignore?
Ignoring requires coordination if there is more than one caregiver involved.
You may also require the cooperation of older children to ignore a younger child.
Ignoring a behaviour for the first time will probably lead to it getting worse before it
    gets better, as your child tries harder to get your negative attention.
Try to distract your child onto something you would rather she did.
Praise her as soon as possible after she starts doing this alternative activity.
With two or more children, pay attention to the child who is doing what you want and
    ignore the child who is doing something you don't want.

Consequences

Natural and logical consequences are a useful behavioural technique, particularly for children of five and over, as they give children more responsibility and help develop decision-making, independence and the ability to learn from mistakes.

Natural consequences consist of leaving things to take their natural course. Examples include allowing a child to get cold if she refuses to put her coat on, or letting a child stay in wet shoes for half an hour if he jumps in a puddle.

Logical consequences are designed by parents to fit the misbehaviour. Examples include: felt tips being removed for half an hour if they are used to draw on walls; locking a bicycle up for 24 hours if it is used on a dangerous road.

There are several *guidelines* to follow for consequences.

➤ Consequences should be appropriate for the age and level of understanding of the child.

➤ Parents should be able to live with the consequences they have chosen, so that they can follow through with them. For example, there is little point in threatening to take the child to school in pyjamas for not getting dressed in time in the morning if this is too embarrassing to do.

➤ Children should be warned in advance of consequences, and whenever possible involved in deciding what is appropriate. For instance, if children are fighting over which television programme to watch, a parent might give them a choice of taking turns to choose the programme, or taking turns not to watch at all.

➤ Consequences should be applied immediately, and not for too long. Persisting too long with a consequence can make it aversive, and consequently less effective (not more effective, as some parents suppose).

➤ Consequences should be applied in a respectful and non-punitive way. For example, washing a child's mouth out with soap for swearing is likely to make him feel degraded and angry. It is also an unacceptable punishment and should be thoroughly discouraged.

➤ Consequences should quickly be followed by an opportunity to carry out the desired behaviour – for instance, once the bicycle or the felt-tips are returned.

A *loss of privilege* is an example of a negative consequence: something that a child would expect to happen is not allowed to happen the next time: for instance (at the evening mealtime): 'If you throw your food on the floor, you won't be allowed to watch the football match'. Of course, this will work only for a child who really wants to watch this particular programme. It is important to generate positive consequences as well as negative ones, as shown in Box 13.16.

A *punishment* is different from a consequence. Although both consequences and time-out (*see* next section) are sometimes construed as forms of punishment, they are far less likely to be effective if they are carried out in a punitive way – rather they should be carried out calmly in a planned way that has (if possible) been agreed with the child in advance, or that can at least be explained to the child as making sense. In contrast, a punishment is a negative, aversive response that is usually carried out impulsively, with anger or irritation. Examples include a smack, toys thrown in the bin or stickers removed from a reward chart. Punishment, despite its reputation (amongst some adults) as the bulwark of child behaviour management, is generally not only ineffective but actually counterproductive. It models the very type of behaviour that most parents would like to see less frequently, and is liable to stoke attitudes in the child of resentment, distrust and low self-esteem: a child may not only become angry at the perceived injustice of an unheralded punishment, but also less likely to agree to do what he is asked.

BOX 13.15 Practice Points about consequences

A natural consequence is what would happen naturally.

A logical consequence fits the behaviour.

A loss of privilege is the removal of something the child expects and desires.

Involve children as much as possible in deciding about consequences and explaining what will happen.

A consequence should follow the behaviour it relates to as quickly as possible.

Consequences are most effective if brief.

Mix positive consequences with negative.

After a negative consequence, find an opportunity for positive interaction, such as praise, as soon as possible.

Avoid punishments if possible.

The case example in Box 13.16 shows a variety of the above techniques, and also illustrates parental problem-solving (*see* below). Daniel is positively reinforced for getting to bed without a fuss by a logical consequence that follows from his agreeing to the television being turned off in time. The logical consequence develops into a reward programme.

BOX 13.16 Continuation of previous case example from Boxes 13.7, 13.9 and 13.13

In session seven, the Family Link worker and Fiona discuss a situation that Fiona has struggled with at home the previous week: Daniel complains vociferously when she turns off the television at 7 pm, and Fiona shouts at him to get up to bed. She tells the Family Link worker she would really like to keep things calm at bedtime.

Together they brainstorm what Fiona could do differently. The suggestions they came up with include the following.

- Telephone Daniel's father, who lives a mile away, to come round and 'sort him out'. The Family Link worker says she would rather Fiona learnt how to sort this out herself, and Fiona agrees.
- Warn Daniel 10 minutes and five minutes before it is time to turn off the television.
- Turn the process into a game, perhaps by racing Daniel upstairs. Fiona does not think this she would be able to run fast enough to make this work!
- Find some other way to distract Daniel, for instance by playing a game with him after the television is turned off. Fiona is worried that this would excite him too much before bedtime and allow things to go on too late.
- Ignore him when he complains or shouts or tantrums.
- Reward him for getting upstairs quickly, for instance by reading him more pages of his storybook, or a short extra story.
- Take a minute off Daniel's story time for every minute he delays.

Fiona says she will try as many of these as she feels comfortable with over the following week, and report back on progress to Helen in the next session.

In session eight, Fiona tells the Family Link worker that Daniel initially made a fuss over all these new rules, as he called them, but Fiona ignored this. Instead she gave a full explanation to Daniel of what they would now do at bedtime. She took Daniel to the library, where they chose some books together so that they were stories he really wanted to hear her read to him. The books Daniel chose became an adequate incentive: after repeated warnings of what would happen next, Daniel earned his extra story on five nights out of seven; on two nights, Helen had to take two minutes off Daniel's story time.

Time-out

Time-out is a shortening of 'time out from positive social reinforcement'. The principle is that bad behaviour is often maintained by any form of social attention, which is rewarding for the child. The behaviour should stop if the attention is removed from the child, either by ignoring, or by all other people in the room leaving it, or by removing the child from the room to an environment where she does not receive any attention. Like many of the other techniques described, time-out requires attention to detail. It is likely to be most successful if started when the child is young (two to five years old), and if there is a positive relationship between the child and parent. This is why play and praise should be taught first. It is best thought of as an opportunity to calm down rather than a punishment: the more of a punishment it becomes, the less likely it is to work.

Time-out is **not suitable for all** children or all parents. Children who are very insecurely attached may become more anxious in response to time-out, so that instead of having the intended calming effect, time-out makes the child more emotionally overwrought, and her behaviour becomes even worse. Children who have been traumatised or abused in the past may experience time-out as abusive, however well it is meant. Some parents use time-out in an excessively punitive way. In all these circumstances, it is probably best not to use time-out, but to rely on other measures, such as ignoring and consequences.

Older children may be able to give themselves time-out, in the sense that they can take themselves to a place where they are able to calm down. This may be their own room, or it may be a space outside the family house. Such self-management should be strongly encouraged.

The choice of a **location** for time-out is crucial. A home visit by the involved professional may be particularly helpful in understanding the possibilities of a particular house or flat. With younger children, time-out can be done successfully with a chair, on the stairs, or in a room. The chair must be in the corner of a room or in a hall, providing this is away from family activities and not in view of the television. Halfway up the stairs can be suitably unstimulating. Some children will not stay on a chair or the step of the stairs, and for these a room is needed, either as a back up or as the first option. The room should preferably be dull and boring, but safe for the child to be alone in. Families with little space may need to use the child's own room for time-out. There are two disadvantages to this – if the child is able to play with or destroy toys or games, these will have to be removed; and if the child finds the experience too aversive, this may make bedtimes more difficult. The name chosen for the time-out place is also important. Calling it the 'naughty step' or the 'bad-boy chair' is implicitly derogatory of the child and indirectly punitive. A more positive name is needed, such as: the 'quiet step', the 'thinking chair', 'having a quiet time to calm down', or just 'time-out'.

Ask a parent to make **two lists of behaviours**: those she would like to see more of and those she would like to see less. It is easier to encourage the positive behaviours first, using praise or tangible rewards. The undesirable behaviours may reduce as the desirable ones increase. Only after this is it worth tackling some of those on the list of unwanted behaviours. Help the parent select *one or two* with which to start time-out. Behaviours which can't be ignored are good ones to choose, such as hitting, sibling fights or being destructive. Non-compliance can also be followed by time-out. Other behaviours can be added after several weeks. The parent should describe to the child what time-out will be like in advance of using it, at a time when the child is calm and receptive (not in the heat of a disciplinary exchange).

The *length* of time-out is also an important consideration. A rough guideline is that the duration should be a minute for each year of age. Durations of longer than five minutes are no more effective than five minutes, and may be counterproductive or even abusive if continued for too long. It can be helpful to set a kitchen timer. Some textbooks suggest the child should be quiet before being let out, but in practice this is not essential. The child needs to get a message that being quiet will get time-out to stop: even a brief period of calm may be sufficient for this. If this does not happen, then alternatives should be tried (*see* below). If time-out works, then it will not need to be used very often, and can be administered for brief periods of five minutes or less, followed immediately by an opportunity for the child to be successful and reap praise.

Time-out can be used for infringements of household rules, such as hitting, or after a *warning* for non-compliance. This will be of the 'if/then' sort: 'If you don't pick that chewing gum up off the floor, then you'll go to time-out'. The warning can be followed by a pause of about five seconds, which can be marked by counting from one to five.

Children may *refuse to go* to time-out. Parents should be advised to *take* children of five and under to time-out, gently but firmly. A child of six years and older should instead have a warning about either going to time-out, losing a privilege, or having some other consequence. This might be, for example, not watching a favourite television programme, or having no access to a favourite games console for a day.

During time-out, most children will at first try to *argue* or wriggle their way out of it. It is important to sustain the child in the time-out setting without getting into an argument, which of course is just another form of gratifying attention. (The parent should, if possible, avoid all interaction during time-out.) Advise the parent to return the child gently to time-out, stating the rule only once more: 'You have to stay in your chair/room for five minutes – you can come out then or earlier if you're quiet'. If the child gets off the chair repeatedly, then a room must be used. The door does not need to be completely shut, and leaving it slightly ajar may help insecure or anxious children to tolerate the procedure. For a child who repeatedly tries to leave the room, the parent will have to shut the door. For children who repeatedly try to open the door, the parent will need to hold the door shut (out of sight of the child). You will have to tailor the procedure to some extent to the particular family. Loss of privilege can also be used as a sanction; for instance: 'If you come out again before the time is up, you won't be able to watch your favourite TV programme tonight'.

Once time-out is over, parents must be calm and positive. If the time-out was for non-compliance, the parent can repeat the original command, which could potentially lead to the whole sequence being repeated (*see* Figure 13.4). The danger of not repeating the command is that some children may use time-out as a means of getting out of chores. However, the parent may decide this would be too aggravating for the child. If so, or if the time out was for behaviours such as hitting,

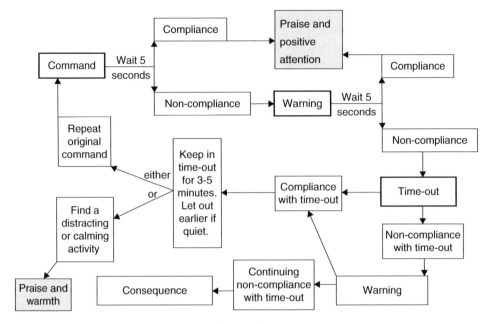

FIGURE 13.4 Sequence of actions in time out

sibling fights or being destructive, the calmness may best be preserved by finding an engrossing or distracting activity for the child.

Parents may themselves need time-out, particularly if feeling stressed, exhausted or emotional. There is a danger that the parent may express too much anger, which may undermine the success of the procedure. The parent must try to conceal any feelings of impatience or frustration and suppress any temptation to criticise, and instead find something as soon as possible to praise. Saying, for instance, (angrily): 'I wish you would play quietly with your sister; you're such a pain when you hit her all the time', while it may be honest, may encourage the child to have a negative view of himself and could also draw attention to the behaviour and make it more likely to happen again. It would probably be more effective to say: 'I know Chloe can be irritating, but that doesn't mean you need to get cross with her', or 'Please can you play separately until you can play together nicely', or wait until they *are* next playing nicely together and then praise them both. The parent may need some professional support to be able to frame what she says constructively.

Parents need specific coaching to *edit out criticisms* and expressions of anger and upset, however understandable these may be. Shouting 'I'm fed up with you messing up the carpet. You make so much extra work. Go to time-out at once!' reflects what most parents must have felt at some time, but is likely to result in the child refusing to go to time-out, or trading insults with the parent, which could lead to an escalating row. Explain to parents that they may need to do some work with their thoughts called 'editing', which involves putting to one side the negative comments they feel like making and instead showing how assertive their calm side can be. You could call it 'acting'. The parent might convert the above situation to an internal dialogue, and say out loud only: 'I warned you that you would have to go to time-out if you didn't pick the chewing gum off the carpet. Now you will have to go. Please get onto the time-out chair'.

Children have a variety of ways of **trying to evade** the isolation of time-out. Some children make a lot of mess. If possible, things that can be messed should be tidied away in advance from the time-out space. Failing this, the child should be expected to tidy his mess after he has calmed down, probably with some parental help. If there are any breakages, a token amount of pocket money could be subtracted from the weekly allowance. Another ploy for getting out of time-out is to threaten not to love the parent any more. Most parents are unaffected by this, but some may give in to reassure their child or themselves: they may need professional support and rehearsal to show no reaction to this.

Parents sometimes say that they think **smacking** is more effective than time-out, because it stops the behaviour more quickly, and punishes the child more effectively. It may be morally right to say that on no account should children be smacked. At the time of writing, smacking is illegal in Scotland but not in England, Wales or Northern Ireland. If you think that the smacking is sufficiently frequent and severe to constitute a safeguarding issue, then you may decide to make a referral to social services. There is however a danger in being judgmental: it may make a parent feel you don't understand how difficult her child is; or it may inhibit the parent from being honest with you about the times she has smacked. Rather than being critical of smacking, it is probably more helpful to discuss smacking and time-out as two alternative strategies, and list the advantages and disadvantages of each, leaving parents to make up their own minds. Our experience is that in general, smacking is ineffective: many children are undeterred by parental threats such as: 'Do you want a smack?' Some parents insist that smacking or threats of physical punishment are effective, although many admit that the main benefit is in relieving their own anger. While smacking may achieve some benefits for the parent in the short-term, it has long-term disadvantages. One is that children learn by modelling that aggression is the way to solve problems and cope with frustration. A second is that children may learn to conceal their actions from their parents, and misbehave more elsewhere than at home. A third is that children may get a message from smacking, and the emotions that go with it, that they are unloved and unlovable, and then live up to this self-image (this may also happen with insults or threats of rejection from parents).

Be sure to safeguard against time-out being used in an **abusive** way. One danger is of its being used for too long. Excessively frequent use can also be dangerous. If not actually abusive, many time-outs in a day are liable to breed resentment, or make children feel they can't do anything right. Ideally, time-out should not be used in a punitive way, but merely as a means of coping with an otherwise out-of-control situation. Most children dislike time-out, but some will learn to take themselves to their room, on their own initiative, to calm down.

Time-out can be used **in public**, for instance outside a supermarket in a corner unobserved by others; or by saying: 'If you continue whining/shouting/tantruming, then you'll have a time-out when you get home'. Of course, this is effective only if followed through at home.

The practice points in Box 13.17 should be read with Figure 13.4.

BOX 13.17 Practice Points for time-out

Use time-out for behaviours that cannot be ignored, or for non-compliance with commands.

Start using it, if at all, under the age of five years.

Don't use it too often.

Plan which space you will use for time-out, and the duration, in advance.

Decide on a positive name for this place.

Give a warning, then wait five seconds to see if the child stops the undesirable behaviour, or starts to comply with your command.

Tell your child to go to the space for the number of minutes you have decided (preferably no more than five).

If she will not comply, carry her if small enough or warn a loss of privilege or negative consequence if not.

Try to pretend to be calm even if you don't feel it: showing how much you are wound up may inadvertently reward your child and encourage her misbehaviour.

Once she is in time-out, ignore your child's attempts to argue, and gently return her if she leaves.

After time-out is over, either find a distracting activity, or repeat the original command.

Find an opportunity as soon as possible for praise and warmth.

If your child will not comply with the command after time-out, you may have to go through the whole cycle again.

BOX 13.18 Continuation of previous Case Example from Box 13.11

The Family Support worker asks the primary mental health worker's advice about how she should help Mike's mother, Juliette, give him time-out. Firstly, they establish that mother and child have a relatively good relationship, which has improved since Mike's sleep routine got better. Secondly, Juliette is in Isabel's opinion very caring, so she would be relatively unlikely to use time-out in an abusive way. Thirdly, the family support worker does not think that Mike has significant attachment insecurity, such as would make him experience time-out as scary or rejecting. So they agree that if Juliette wants to try time-out, then the family support worker should help her.

The primary mental health worker and the family support worker discuss the above outline of time-out, emphasising the need to choose which behaviours Juliette wants to tackle, how the Family Support Worker can help her decide where to put Mike for four minutes, how Juliette would be able to keep him there, and how she could remain calm throughout and be positive with him as soon as possible afterwards.

Two weeks later, the family support worker reports that Juliette has chosen to sit Mike halfway up the stairs, as she thinks this would be a suitably un-stimulating place. She has however found it difficult to keep him there, and unfortunately got into an argument with him about it, which rather defeated the objective of time-out.

The family support worker and the primary mental health worker brainstorm solutions to this. They think about asking Juliette to put Mike on a time-out chair in a corner of the most boring room in the house, but it is not a very large house, and it would be difficult to stop Mike's two-year-old sister from trying to play with him or perhaps trying to wind him up. They agree to try to get Mike into his room and keep him there. The family support worker suggests holding the door shut, but the primary mental health worker is uncomfortable with this and suggests that Juliette should return Mike to his room, calmly and neutrally, as often as it takes for him to get the message that he should stay there. Juliette will need to explain to Mike that he needs to sit and be calm before he can come out.

Two weeks later, Isabel reports that Juliette has tried this three times. The first time, Mike made a big fuss, but became slightly calmer at the end of the four minutes. Juliette thought of a game to play with both children when the time-out period was finished, and she managed to make this into an enjoyable experience, so she could get in some smiles and hugs. The second time, Mike complained less about having to go to his room, and by the third time, he went to his room in a resigned way, and come out a lot calmer after the four minutes were over.

Problem-solving

Many parents of children with behaviour problems have deficits in problem-solving skills, and this is known to be a significant factor in adolescent conduct disorder. Problem-solving tuition can be done for both parents and young children (given time), using the following five steps:

➤ define the problem: What am I supposed to do?
➤ brainstorm solutions: What are some plans?
➤ evaluate consequences: What is the best plan?
➤ implementation: Am I using my plan?
➤ evaluating the outcome and revising the plan: How did I do?

Younger children may have difficulty with the last two steps, but can consider several alternative solutions, and can understand that some are better than others.

Parents can be helped to teach children problem-solving with the use of stories, puppets and cartoons. Firstly, parents can discuss hypothetical problems and go through the five steps. Secondly, they can use the techniques for real-life problems. It is then important for the parent to establish the child's view of the problem before coming to her own conclusions; then to help the child generate solutions, however daft; then to look at the consequences of the most promising two or three; then to help the child try out one or two. Parents may need help with their own feelings before being able to help their child think about her feelings, and about the feelings of other people in the problem situation. The aim is to encourage the process of problem-solving, not necessarily to arrive first time at the best solution.

BOX 13.19 Case Example

> Louise feels devastated that her four-year-old son, Kevin, has been sent home early from a friend's house because he got into a fight. She decides to find out what happened, both from her son and his friend's parent, and then discuss what could happen differently next time. She starts by trying to understand Kevin's point of view. Kevin's friend said he didn't think Kevin had any good DVDs, and Kevin overreacted to this by hitting.
>
> They talk about what he could do the next time somebody says something he doesn't like. Various solutions come up in the discussion: to go home, to say something nasty back, to steal one of his friend's DVDs or to kick him harder than before. Louise explores his feelings further by asking, 'How are you feeling about being sent home?' 'How did you feel when he said that about your DVDs?' and helps Kevin think about his friend's feelings. She asks, 'How do you think he felt when you hit him?' 'How can you tell if he is sad or happy?' 'What would happen if you said something nasty to him?' 'What would happen if you stole one of his DVDs?' 'How can you make him be your friend?' Eventually Kevin says that his friend asked to borrow a toy of his and, with a little help from his mother, comes up with the idea of offering to swap this toy for one of his friend's DVDs.

BOX 13.20 Practice Points for problem-solving

> What exactly is the problem?
> Think of as many solutions as possible, however daft some of them may seem.
> Choose one or two to try.
> How did it go?
> If one did not work, try another one.
> What did you learn?

What to do if you lose it

Parents may feel guilty if they shout at their children, as professional advice usually suggests shouting is a 'bad thing'. Frequent shouting is likely to very much diminish its own effectiveness. Most children are resilient enough to cope with being shouted at occasionally, but one possible danger of being shouted is a lowering of self-esteem. Some children may try really hard to wind a parent up. So it may be worth rehearsing with a parent how she thinks she could recover the situation after a child gets under her skin.

One option might be to give the child a hug. Once the child and parent are calm, it may be helpful for the parent to explain what made her so cross. Some parents may be able to apologise for getting too cross; to others this may feel inappropriate. Others may feel able to explain when they get easily irritated that there is a particular worry or emotional upset that has contributed to this. Young children can be very good at accepting these sorts of explanation, providing they are couched in age-appropriate language. Some such way of re-establishing emotional warmth may serve to restore the respect between parent and child.

A word on exercise

Cultural norms in the 21st century do not necessarily encourage exercise as a part of everyday life. Children may be driven to school and not allowed outside to play, due to lack of safe space. Home activities may be dominated by console games, use of a personal computer, television or passive watching of other media (such as DVDs). Therefore the only exercise some children have may be in twice-weekly physical education lessons. In addition to increasing the risk of obesity, this is likely to make children's behaviour more difficult to manage. Some of the content that children watch may encourage aggressive behaviour. Parents may find the behaviour of their children easier to cope with if they can find ways of getting their children to have more exercise and less dependence on screen watching (*see* Chapter 44 on Diet and Exercise).

Referral

Within universal services there are usually behaviour management/parenting groups available, which may require professional referral or self-referral. Some may be available only via specialist services.

This chapter has focused on the Webster-Stratton model of behaviour management, which is only one among several. Other models have already been mentioned; an alternative approach to behaviour management integrates it with the psychodynamic ideas of containment and reciprocity.[11] The theoretical basis of the Solihull Approach arose partly out of infant observation, but the practical application involves constructing with the family members who are present a story that enables a fresh understanding of what they see as the problem: this can help them generate their own novel ways of dealing with it.

Referral to specialist CAMHS is not necessarily appropriate as an initial step, but may be discussed later. It may become necessary if it seems likely there is a further condition affecting the child's behaviour that needs assessment, for example ADHD or autistic spectrum disorder.

RESOURCES

Books for parents on behaviour management

- Byron T. *The House of Tiny Tearaways*. London: BBC Active; 2005.
  Although derived from a television series, this book gives sensible and practical suggestions, and examples of how to make them work, for children aged one to seven years.
- Early Support. *Information for Parents: behaviour*. London: Department for Children, Schools and Families; 2010.
- Eastman M. *Taming the Dragon in Your Child: solutions for breaking the cycle of family anger*. Chichester: John Wiley; 1994.
  This book gives advice on helping children aged one to 16 years (and their parents) manage their angry feelings.

- Jayson D. *Understanding Children's Behaviour*. 2nd ed. London: Family Doctor Publications (British Medical Association); 2008.
  If a child (infant to pre-teenager) is difficult to manage, this book offers some strategies to try.
- Faber A, Mazlish E. *How to Talk So Kids Will Listen and Listen So Kids Will Talk*. UK: Piccadilly Press; 2001.
- Green C, Roberts R. *New Toddler Taming: a parent's guide to the first four years*. London: Vermillion; 2001.
  This book is full of practical advice on how to deal with common toddler problems and difficult behaviour.
- Greene RW. *The Explosive Child: a new approach for understanding and parenting easily frustrated, chronically inflexible children*. 2nd ed. London: HarperPaperbacks; 2010.
- Hunt C. *The Parenting Puzzle: how to get the best out of family life*. London: Family Links; 2003. For ages one to seven years, this book, linked to a 10-week behaviour management course called the 'Nurturing Programme', addresses feelings as well as behaviours for children and parents.
- Phelan T. *1-2-3 Magic: effective discipline for children 2-12*. 4th ed. Illinois: ParentMagic, Incorporated; 2010.
  This guide for carers offers behavioural advice for managing common child behaviour problems.
- Sullivan K. *How to Say No and Mean It*. 2nd ed. London: Thorsons; 2005.
- Webster-Stratton C. *The Incredible Years*. Seattle, WA: The Incredible Years; 2006.
  This book is linked to one of the most evidence-based parenting programmes and gives advice on managing behavioural difficulties and parenting strategies for children aged three to eight years.

Websites

- Mumsnet: This website hosts loads of information and views of interest to parents. www. mumsnet.com
- Netmums: This site provides local listings for dads as well as mums. www.netmums.com
- Family Lives: This website provides tips for anyone caring for any age of child. http:// familylives.org.uk
- Some other websites are included in the reference list below.

REFERENCES

1 National Institute for Health and Clinical Excellence. NICE technology appraisal guidance 102: Parent-training/education programmes in the management of children with conduct disorders. London: National Institute for Health and Clinical Excellence; 2006. Available at: www.nice.org.uk/TA102 or www.scie.org.uk/publications/children.asp (accessed 26 March 2011).
2 Lexmond J, Reeves R. *Building Character*. London: Demos; 2009. Available at: www.demos. co.uk/files/Building_Character_Web.pdf?1257752612 (accessed 26 March 2011). In: Marmot M. *Fair Society, Healthy Lives: strategic review of health inequalities in England post-2010* [Marmot review final report]. London: University College; 2010. p. 99.
3 www.incredibleyears.com
4 www.mellowparenting.org
5 www.parentsplus.ie

6 www.triplep.net
7 www.commissioningtoolkit.org
8 www.parentlink.org.uk
9 National Institute for Health and Clinical Excellence, op. cit.
10 Figures 13.2 and 13.3 are loosely based on diagrams in: Patterson GR, Reid JB, Dishion TJ. *Antisocial Boys.* Eugene, Oregon: Castalia; 1992.
11 www.solihull.nhs.uk/solihullapproach

Index